# Amazing Courage

## My Life as a Polio Survivor

**Margy Dieguez**

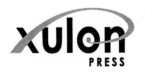
**xulon** PRESS

www.xulonpress.com

*This book is dedicated to
my son Robert and my daughter Renee*

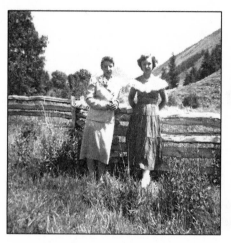

*Mary Jo and Margaret Ann*

Two sisters who have shared a bond even deeper
than the natural bond of family.

# *Acknowledgments*

My story begins when I was fifteen years old. On August 7, 1952, I was diagnosed with polio, the dreaded disease the entire United States feared. It was two years before the vaccine was discovered by Jonas Salk.

Many times I have been asked, "What exactly is your disability?" and when I tell them I had polio, many have responded with, "You need to write a book." Throughout the years, my friends and family, too, have tried to persuade me to write the story of my life.

I wasn't sure how to begin or what to say until I read a book by my friend and coworker from the College of the Canyons, Rosemarie Walrath. Her book, *My Two Sons,* chronicles her life with her two sons who have muscular dystrophy. Her own effort at writing and willingness to share her story encouraged me to write my own.

I have many, many friends who have encouraged me and helped me throughout my life. During the last eleven years, my caregivers have helped preserve my independence, and I am very grateful to them for that.

Sherry Ragan has been my caregiver and friend for the last seven of those years, but I have had so very many others, such as Connie, Sally, Maria, Gloria, Diane and Felicia They have all enriched my life in innumerable ways. Chris Dimwidde was not only my caregiver but also my consultant as together we went page by page through my manuscript.

A special thanks to Brenda Pitts for her formatting and editing of my manuscript. She took my words and with professionalism and flair brought my story to life. I'm thankful to have found her exceptional editorial service.

My story is the story of a woman who had to find a way to overcome everyday problems posing monumental obstacles. It is my belief that my life has been what it was supposed to be. With the love and support of my son, Robert, and my daughter, Renee, coupled with my belief in God, I have lived life to the fullest. For that, I am forever grateful for all the amazing people who helped me along the way and the amazing God who made it all possible.

# *Chapter 1*

*T*he heat waves shimmered off the highway on the road ahead. Not only the searing sun but also the oppressive humidity made it hard for me to catch my breath. It was the summer of 1952, and my parents, my sister and her young son, and I were driving through the Midwest on our way home from California. It was so terribly hot, and as we passed through a town in Kansas, I longingly watched a group of people cooling off in a swimming pool.

"Daddy, please, let's stop and swim," I begged. "I'm so hot, and it wouldn't take too long. Could we please?"

"No, Dad answered. "I know you're hot, but it's August, you know. And that means polio time. We'll just stop and get a block of ice to put on the floor in the backseat. That'll cool you off."

I sighed heavily, knowing he had made up his mind. The block of ice would have to do. We finally made it home to Warrensburg, and the cool breeze wafting through the house was a wonderful relief.

We had brought my sister, Mary Jo, who was pregnant with her second child, home for a visit before the baby was born. I was glad to have her and my nephew with us, but it had been a long, hot trip to get them and then return home.

I was fifteen years old that summer and would soon begin my freshman year in high school, a very big deal to me. To my great joy, I had been selected as one of six cheerleaders, and we were having summer practices. I could hardly wait to assume my cheerleading position and all the excitement and bustle sure to accompany it.

During my years in school, I had always participated in lots of extracurricular activities. I had taken baton lessons for years, and in the eighth grade, I was privileged to be one of the majorettes leading the band in parades down the main street of our town. In junior high, I was even elected princess of our annual school dance. I relished all the flurry of activity that was part of my life and eagerly anticipated all that was to come with my advancement to high school.

A few days after getting home from California, both my sister and I got very sick. I had a fever and sore throat, and Mary Jo had chills and a bad headache. On Friday the family doctor decided both of us should be admitted to the hospital so we could be watched.

Mary Jo and I were in the same hospital room, and we talked about an article she had read in a magazine that discussed the virus running rampant throughout the United States at that time. Technically called infantile paralysis, the dreaded virus was more commonly known as polio. There had been sixty thousand documented cases and three thousand deaths that year, the last big epidemic before Dr. Jonas Salk discovered his vaccine.

"Mary Jo, do you think maybe that's what's wrong with us?" I asked worriedly. "Do you think maybe we have polio, like all those other people?"

Mary Jo seemed reluctant to answer. After a brief silence, she responded, "Well . . . it's possible, I guess. Our symptoms are like what I read, and we do feel bad enough. Maybe we do have polio . . . but then again, maybe we don't," she hastily added.

Monday morning soon arrived. I felt so much better that the doctor let me go home. Since my sister was pregnant, he felt she should be monitored a while longer. By Wednesday my mother was growing quite upset with the doctor because he still had not diagnosed the problem with my sister. Finally, they performed a spinal tap on her, and the results were devastating: Mary Jo had polio. She was immediately whisked away by ambulance to General Hospital in Kansas City and put in the isolation ward.

From Monday until Friday of that week, I filled my time with babysitting for Donnie, Mary Jo's son, pulling weeds in the front yard, and roller skating at the local rink. In those days, I was quite a tomboy, playing football, climbing trees, and playing cowboys and Indians. So I found plenty of ways to keep myself busy and to keep my mind off the tragedy that had befallen our family.

But in a small town such as ours, one family's misfortune touches everyone else. My parents, respected members of the community, owned a flower shop and several greenhouses in town, but after word of Mary Jo's diagnosis spread, people began avoiding us. Many were so terrified of catching polio from us that they would walk on the opposite side of the street from our business to minimize contact with us.

In all fairness to the townspeople, it must be said that at that time no one knew exactly how polio was contracted. All anyone knew was that it was a horrible disease that struck without warning and showed no respecter of persons. Everyone was affected by the disease either directly or indirectly. The owner of the drugstore in town suffered the loss of two children. A young boy I went to church with also died. These were just two of the many deaths resulting from the dreaded disease.

The fear generated by polio was almost as para-lyzing as the illness itself. Desperate measures were taken to try to hold the sickness at bay. Streets were sprayed with a disinfectant, theaters closed their doors, and although churches continued their services, fewer people attended. With fear running rampant, our safe, happy little town became virtually a ghost town.

On the following Friday after I had come home from the hospital, I got up to go to the bathroom but had trouble walking. My parents were frantic. One of their precious daughters already had polio, and now it looked as though the other one might have it too. Nearly beside themselves with worry, my parents immediately contacted the doctor, who came to the house to do a spinal tap. The result—just like it had been with Mary Jo—was devastating: I, too, had polio. According to the doctor, I actually had a mild case of the disease, but because I had been so active during the previous week, the virus had done a great deal of damage.

There are defining moments that occur in all our lives, and my diagnosis of polio was mine. I remember my dad sitting at the kitchen table and crying for hours. Heartbroken, he now had to deal with the fact that both of his daughters were ravaged by the same cruel disease. His life, my mother's life, Mary Jo and her family's life, and my life were all changed forever in that one moment in the summer of 1952.

# *Chapter 2*

*T* was immediately transported by ambulance to the same hospital where Mary Jo was staying. The first thing I noticed upon entering was a contraption called an iron lung. Although this type of medical equipment is seldom used today, it played a crucial role in saving lives during the peak of the polio epidemic in the 1950s.

The iron lung consisted of a long metal cylinder enclosing all of a person's body except for the head, which rested on a platform just outside the cylinder. As the iron lung "breathed" for the patient, a distinctive whooshing sound of the life-giving care being rendered was emitted. This is the sound that greeted me as I entered the hospital that day.

Soon I was taken to a room to be with my sister. She greeted me warmly, but concern filled her eyes. "Oh, I'm so glad to see you, but I wish you didn't have to be here. Are you okay, Margy?" Mary Jo asked, always the big sister.

"Yeah, I'm okay, I guess," I answered slowly. I was not happy to be there, but I have always been the stoic type and do not recall being overly agitated at that moment about my condition. We chatted for a while, two sisters sharing a bond even deeper than the natural bond of family.

After I had been in the room for several hours, I was suddenly aroused from my thoughts by the distressed voice of my big sister. "Nurse, nurse! I need a nurse!" Mary Jo frantically called. The nurse on duty flew into the room, and Mary Jo, her voice breaking, said, "I'm . . . I'm . . . having contractions. It's too early. . . It's not time yet. . . Oh, please, I don't want to lose this baby!" The nurse did her best to calm Mary Jo and then whisked her away to another room.

Despite everyone's best efforts, Mary Jo did miscarry. The baby was lost and the priest called in to baptize it. Now, on top of the polio, Mary Jo had to contend with the grief and sorrow of losing her child.

Hearing the news, her husband flew in from California to be with her, but he wasn't even allowed into the isolation ward to see his wife. He and my parents had to stand helplessly outside and try to communicate with her and me through a window. By this point, I was not able to roll myself onto my side, so the nurses did it for me and propped me up with pillows so that I could look out the window.

Soon I began to experience some difficulty in breathing, and when this was brought to the doctor's attention, he announced, "I'm going to make a little hole in your throat to help you breathe better." Unknown to me at the time, this surgical procedure is called a tracheotomy and opens a direct airway through an incision in the neck into the windpipe. My throat was deadened for the procedure, but I could feel the pressure as they cut.

Lying there, helpless and vulnerable, I heard one doctor speak as though he was issuing orders: "Don't cut here . . . go there . . . do it this way."

That scared me, and I asked in a trembling voice, "Are you experimenting on me? Are you sure you know what you're doing Not until years later did I realize that the hospital was a teaching hospital, but at the time, all I knew was that I was frightened.

Looking around desperately, I caught the attention of one of the nurses and begged her, "Please, could you pray with me? I'm so scared!" She kindly took my hand and together we prayed, "Hail Mary, full of grace, the Lord is with thee. Blessed art thou amongst women, and . . ." My words trailed off as the incision was made and the air began escaping through the hole in my neck. Although I continued to move my lips, no sound came out. A curved metal tube was inserted into the hole, and the procedure was quickly finished. Little did I know that it would be five long months before I would again speak naturally.

At least the procedure was over and I could return to the safety and comfort of my room with Mary Jo, I thought. But instead of taking me back to the room with my sister, I was transferred to a very large room in the basement of the hospital. It was the iron lung room! Panicked, I started to cry because I was so afraid they would put my head as well as my body into the cylindrical tube.

As they moved me from the gurney to the lung, my head fell limply backward. That in itself was terrifying enough, but my fear greatly intensified when I discovered I couldn't lift it back up on my own. At that point, I realized the awful truth: I was totally paralyzed. Fifteen years old, with all my future before me, and I couldn't even lift my own head. My usual stoicism crumbled as I considered what all this meant.

As my mind was whirling with so many thoughts, the nurses and attendants were busy positioning me within the iron lung. They laid me flat on my back on a board about eighteen inches wide and then pushed me inside the cylinder. To my great relief, although my entire body was enclosed, my head was not, but rested on a stand outside the lid of the cylinder. A rubber collar padded with soft foam encircled my neck to provide comfort but, even more crucial, to maintain the air pressure inside the cylinder. If air escaped, the pressure would be lost, and I wouldn't be able to breathe. The same foam was used on the holes on the side of the lung where the nurses could reach inside to move me.

A mirror over my head allowed me to see what was happening in the room. That was the only thing I had to relieve the monotony of the endless hours I faced each day. I actually looked forward to each morning before breakfast when I could watch the nurses as they moved from patient to patient. That was my life for the next forty days: flat on my back, enclosed in an iron lung, and completely unable to move.

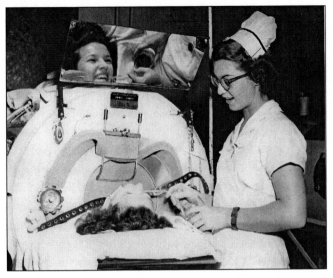

*The iron lung: A drink from my nurse*

On one occasion in those forty days, I did have a break in the monotony—though not the kind of break you would hope for: the electricity in the building went out! Pandemonium and panic erupted throughout the hospital as all the attendants rushed to hand pump all the iron lungs. To their credit and everyone's relief, they performed their duties wonderfully, and no one was harmed. When the power came back on, however, my sister insisted on coming out from her isolation room to see for herself that I was all right. She relentlessly badgered an orderly until he put her in a wheelchair and pushed her out to see me. After such a horrible scare, it was so good for both of us to see each other and know that we were fine.

During my time spent in the iron lung room in the basement, my parents could look at me through a small window in a cutaway area at the base of the building. The nurse would turn my iron lung so I could see them, and I would try to read their lips. This was our only communication during those dark days.

The polio that I had contracted was a severe, debilitating form called paralytic polio. In addition, I suffered from respiratory polio, or bulbospinal polio. With these two dangerous strains of the disease, I could neither move on my own, other than to slightly move my head from side to side, nor breathe on my own. A physical therapist came daily to do range-of-motion exercises so my body would remain flexible. After a week of therapy, I did regain some movement in my right arm and leg, but it's never been normal. To this day, I'm unable to use my left hand at all, and I can't lift either arm over my shoulder. The left leg never regained much movement, so I always wore a leg brace until I became permanently confined to a wheelchair.

At the time, of course, I had no way of knowing the long-lasting effects of the disease on my body. I just took it day by day, trying my best to believe for a better future. I shared my space in the polio isolation basement with many, many others facing the same ordeal and hoping for the same outcome. Crammed together in that room, we were all victims of the same cruel disease.

There were so many patients in the room that the nurses could barely walk between us. The iron lungs were lined up along one wall, baby cribs were along the opposite wall, and beds with patients occupied the middle of the room. The babies didn't cry much—they just whimpered—and I watched as one baby after another died, was wrapped up, and taken away. One night doctors and nurses hovered for hours over the man in the lung next to me. He was gone the next morning.

Soon people all around me were dying. Five days after I arrived, a priest and my parents were allowed to come in to see me so the priest could give me the last sacrament of the Catholic Church, the sacrament for the dying. Each of them was covered from head to toe with a gown and a mask. Being only fifteen years old, I had no idea that I wasn't expected to live, but I'm sure it must have been quite devastating for my parents to have their daughter receive this sacred rite. Even though I didn't fully understand the sacrament and what it meant, it gave me such a wonderful feeling of peace and comfort.

Forty days later, I was finally taken out of the lung. Though I knew this was a necessary part of my recovery, I was extremely apprehensive because I had become dependent on it to breathe for me. I wondered what would happen when my body was expected to resume this function on its own.

Much to my dismay, the first time I was pulled out, I immediately started gasping for air and had to be returned to the lung right away. But they tried again, and this time I was able to stay out for a few minutes. Each day I was able to stay out a little longer. To help with the transition to breathing, the nurses put a shell-like object over me. Called the "turtle," it was strapped to my chest and had the same in-and-out breathing motion as the iron lung.

Gradually, however, I was able to breathe completely on my own. As soon as I was free of the iron lung, I was moved to a private room, although still in isolation. Many of my classmates and friends traveled the fifty miles to the hospital just to see me. Since they were not allowed in my room, they came in groups of three or four and stood outside my window to talk to me. Sometimes it would be snowing, but still they came, stomping their feet and clapping their hands to keep warm. They would talk loudly and make funny faces to make me laugh, brightening my day in so many kind and wonderful ways.

I had gone into isolation on August 7, 1952, but in my youthful optimism, I always expected to be going home soon. My brother was playing football at the Los Angeles Coliseum on Thanksgiving Day, and I planned on making that game. That day came and went, with me, of course, still in the hospital, so I shifted my attention to Christmas. Surely I would make it home for Christmas, I thought. I didn't make it home by Christmas, but I did get out of isolation.

One bright spot in all my troubles was that Mary Jo's recovery was much more rapid. After several weeks in the hospital, she was allowed to return home to California. She had physical therapy for a short time and suffered no severe problems afterward.

Another big event in my hospital stay occurred on December 1 when my tracheotomy tube was finally removed and I was able to talk normally again. I was moved from General Hospital's isolation to St. Luke's Hospital in Kansas City. Thankfully, I could now get out of the hospital bed and into a wheelchair.

After five months of being in an isolation ward, I was overjoyed to be in a regular hospital room. This was a very exciting time for me because now my family and friends could come into my room and visit. And visit they did!

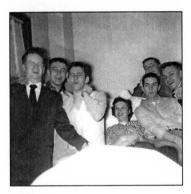

*My visiting high school friends*

Every day after closing the flower shop, my mother drove the fifty miles to the hospital. Even when it was snowing, she still came, never missing a day. I eagerly looked forward to her visit and loved hearing the clickety-click of her high-heeled shoes as she walked down the hallway toward my room. That is one of my fond memories in the midst of so many other difficult ones. As I said, I did not make it home for Christmas, but Christmas certainly made its way to me!

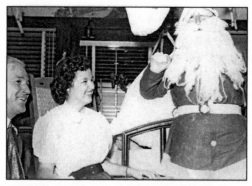

***Celebrating Christmas with my dad and Santa***

I was simply overwhelmed with the outpouring of cards, presents, and expressions of kindness. My bed was piled high with so many gifts, and I let my brother, Joe, open them for me. Caught up in the holiday mood, he opened them so quickly that we never knew who sent what and couldn't send the proper thank-you notes.

A Jesuit priest from Rockhurst College came regularly to my room to help me with my school studies so I could keep up with my class. We spent a lot of time reading and studying English literature. Those sessions with the priest gave me a long-lasting love of literature.

A nun also came to help me, and she said something that made a permanent impression on me. She said, "God must love you very much to let you help Him carry His cross." Those words had an incredible impact on me, both at the time she said them and many times later. Mulling over her words, I have always felt there was a reason that I was allowed to have a lifelong disability. I've come to the conclusion that I am exactly where I'm meant to be, and that acceptance has kept me from any unhappiness or bitterness. Throughout my life, at the times when I most needed it, her words have come back to encourage me and keep me moving forward.

While I was at St. Luke's, a physical therapist began working with me in a wonderful therapeutic pool. With help from the therapist, I actually stood up in the water, much to my great delight. What an incredible feeling to be upright again! Because of the buoyancy of the water, I could move my leg a little, and I let it float up. Then I leaned my body forward and pushed it back down. With the therapist holding on to my side, I took a few steps forward, the first in six months.

# Chapter 3

*A*fter a month at St. Luke's Hospital, I was accepted as a patient at a rehabilitation center in Warm Springs, Georgia. This is the center made famous by President Franklin Roosevelt when he visited the warm mineral springs there. Gushing from the hillside of Pine Mountain at a constant eighty-eight degrees, the water, it was hoped, would strengthen his legs paralyzed from polio. I was very fortunate to be accepted at Warm Springs. There was quite a long waiting list, but my parents knew a doctor who helped gain my acceptance into the program.

Lying on a hospital stretcher, I was transported by ambulance to the Kansas City train terminal for the long ride to Georgia. Mother had reserved a compartment on the train so that I could be in bed for most of the trip; I was still not able to sit up for any length of time. But with her assistance, I made the trip just fine.

The Warm Springs Rehabilitation Center was located on a lovely campus with green lawns and impressive-looking buildings with white colonnades. As I lay on the backseat of the car, I had a unique view of the treetops as we drove through the main entrance. At fifteen years old, I had no idea what was happening to me or what the future would hold, but I felt very secure because I knew my parents would take care of me. I have often thought what a wonderful gift that is for parents to give their children and how fortunate I was to have it.

As a patient at the center, I received water therapy, regular therapy, and occupational therapy once a day. It was very rigorous, a great deal of work, and very, very tiring. But that was the reason I was there, so I did my best to take advantage of all the excellent care and training offered.

I shared a room with three other girls: Shelly, Sheila, and Laurie. We each had our own individual struggles, but I felt especially sorry for Shelly. Shelly was my age; her legs were fine, but her arms and hands were totally paralyzed and completely useless. She could walk up to a door but was unable to open it and walk through it. After she left the center, I heard that she simply sat on her front porch, day after day, very depressed.

Sheila was from Colorado, and later, after being discharged from the center, I visited her. Sheila was working for her father in his drugstore and loving it, busy with life and moving on from the past. Later Mother and I also visited Laurie in Phoenix, Arizona. She had married the man she was engaged to before she contracted polio. Her sister was living with them to take care of her. Sadly, less than a year after we visited, Laurie died from pneumonia.

But back to our life at the center. The foundation operated its own brace shop, where each patient was fitted for the necessary appliances. In my case, my arms and hands had been badly affected by the polio, but I did retain some use of them. So the technicians constructed a hanger frame above my wheelchair with springs coming down from it. My arms were placed in cuffs, and the springs were used to keep my shoulders from coming out of their sockets. This allowed me to move my arms.

For my left leg, a foot-to-thigh brace was fashioned to supplement two crutches. When they stood me up for the first time, I fell over because I had no strength in my back or stomach. To correct this problem, they fitted me with a metal back brace. With the aid of these braces and crutches, I began making progress toward walking again.

My life was set to a rigorous and predictable schedule. There were strengthening exercises in the morning, pool in the early afternoon, and walking in the late afternoon. I did very well and especially looked forward to the walking exercises—well, most of the time! I remember one time in particular when my therapist made me walk up an incline. It was steep and very hard, but she pushed and pushed me to do it. Finally, I got angry, but she still kept pushing me until I cried. She was not to be deterred, however, regardless of my anger or tears. My legs ached and I was exhausted, but she would not let me give up. Because of her tenacity, I eventually made it up the incline, and in that moment, the anger and tears were replaced by feelings of gratitude for her perseverance.

One bright spot in all the rehabilitation was the fact that young men from neighboring schools came to Warm Springs to push the patients and take them to doctor and rehabilitation appointments on the campus. These young men were called "push boys." My roommates and I soon became good friends with three of them: J. R., Burt, and Herb. When the girls and I weren't in therapy, we played cards, listened to music, and had a great time with the boys. Sometimes we had races down the hill in our wheelchairs. Other times the push boys would take us out of our chairs so they could get in them and race down the hill. We had lots of fun and laughs, just like normal teenagers.

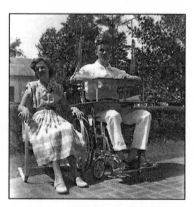

*J.R. and I trading places*

Feeling normal was a big goal for all of us, and the center helped facilitate that feeling. Every morning we started the day by dressing in regular clothes for our daily activities and for going to the main dining room. These small things, coupled with the friendship of the push boys and my physical progress, helped me begin to feel normal again, little by little.

Part of my daily routine was to visit the therapy pool. Here the soothing water from the springs allowed me to move so much more easily. The side of the pool was built three feet high off the walkway, which raised the water level higher than the floor. This design, however, allowed a patient on a gurney to simply slide into the pool without having to be lifted.

As I was slid into the water, the therapist would hold my head and float me over to a slanted wooden table. My head was kept out of the water while the therapist worked with my arms and legs under the water. After seven months of this kind of intense therapy, along with the aid of the leg brace, back brace and two crutches, I was finally able to stand on my own. Taking little steps, I was soon able to walk across a room.

From January until August of 1953, I worked with the therapists at the center. Finally, on August 7, 1953, exactly one year to the day when I had entered the Kansas City General Hospital, I was dismissed from the rehabilitation center and allowed to return home. Both Mom and Dad traveled to Georgia for the big occasion.

I was very excited to be on my way home at last. My dad made a pallet in the back of the station wagon so I could lie down part of the time. We had wonderful plans to celebrate my release, including traveling up the east coast to Washington, D.C. to see the White House, the Capitol, and all the famous monuments.

But it didn't turn out exactly like we had planned. On that first day, we drove into Savannah and stopped at a restaurant for lunch. By now I was very sick with strep throat and couldn't go into the restaurant, so my dad brought soup out to me.

"Here, Margy, try this. Maybe it'll make your throat feel better," Daddy said kindly as he handed me the bowl.

I appreciated his kindness, but I guess he could tell that I was having difficulty swallowing because he soon took the bowl from me and worriedly asked, "What's the matter? Aren't you hungry? Is your throat hurting really bad?"

I nodded, blinking back tears, and he and Mom conferred for a moment before deciding to take me to a doctor. As soon as the doctor saw me, he wanted to put me into the hospital. In a matter-of-fact tone, he announced, "We need to get this young lady into the hospital right away. I don't like the looks of that throat, and with all she's been through, I don't think we can be too careful."

I had just finished a year of hospitals, and I was fiercely against it. Totally out of character for me, I absolutely refused. "No, I will *not* go into another hospital. I am on my way home, and I am going to enjoy every minute of it. It's nothing more than a sore throat, and I'll get over it," I insisted.

Much to my surprise, my parents sided with me and decided we would give my way a try. We left Savannah and drove up to Washington, D.C., and when we got there, my dad rented a limousine so I could at least look out the window at all the famous landmarks. I tried my best to enjoy the sights, but I wasn't getting any better.

Dad and Mom talked again and decided it would be best for Mom and me to fly home to Kansas City. This time I didn't object, but when Dad tried to purchase our tickets, the airline was reluctant to take me aboard. Only after he signed all sorts of papers releasing them from liability did they agree to allow me aboard. In that way, Mom and I made it home, while Daddy drove back to Missouri by himself.

# *Chapter 4*

*I*t was time for another school year to begin.

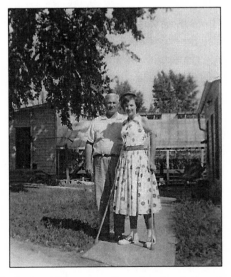

*My dad and I on my first day back to school*

Because of my studies at the school on the Warm Springs campus, I had been able to keep up with my class although I had missed a full year. I was so excited to be returning to school and being with all my friends that I had grown up with. There was a problem, though, that had to be solved: I wasn't able to climb steps, and our high school had a second floor. How was I going to be able to maneuver the steps to get to class?

The boys thought up the perfect solution. Whenever I needed to go upstairs, two boys would grasp each other's arms and make a seat for me to sit on. I would unlatch my brace, sit down, put an arm around each boy's neck, and away we would go! For the next three years, I was carried up and down the stairs in this unique fashion. And thank heaven, there was always someone around willing to help.

My high school was very welcoming and accepting of me. So many people helped me at different times, and I will never forget their kindness. For instance, in my junior year, I was a candidate for homecoming queen. During the parade through town, I had to sit on the back of a convertible. My balance wasn't that great, so two of my friends sat on either side of me and held on to me so I wouldn't fall off. During halftime at the football game that night, I walked out to the middle of the field and was crowned homecoming queen. What a moment—not only to be selected queen but also to walk out onto the football field to claim the honor! I had come a long way in a year, and a lot of people had helped me get there.

Later at the homecoming dance, the teachers and students waited as my date, a boy named Holmes, and I led the first dance.

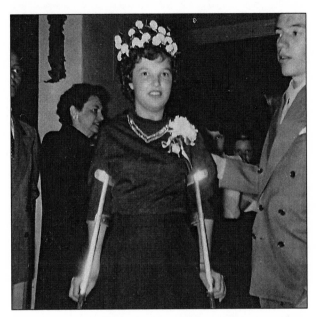

***Leading the Homecoming Dance***

I leaned my crutches against the wall and held on to Holmes as we walked to the middle of the gym. I was a little nervous until the band started to play. But Holmes held on to me firmly, and once we started dancing, I was fine. This was just one of so many ordinary occurrences that were extraordinary for me. Polio had changed everything, and I couldn't take for granted the simple things that most people never even think about.

Another one of those landmark ordinary occurrences happened that same year. My dad and I were in Kansas City when he suddenly decided to buy a new car. We went to a Buick dealer, and he bought a station wagon. On the highway on our way home to Warrensburg, he suddenly pulled off to the side of the road and startled me by saying, "Okay, Margy, it's your turn now. Get behind the wheel and drive."

"But, Daddy, I don't know if I can. I don't think I'm strong enough to handle the steering wheel," I protested.

"That's the beauty of these new cars," My dad explained. "They have power steering, so it's really easy to drive them. Come on and give it a try, Margy. You can do it."

I was quite nervous, but like any young girl, I did want to drive. I climbed behind the wheel and was amazed at how easy it was. My right foot was strong enough to use the gas and brake pedals, and with the power steering, I could maneuver the steering wheel as well. Dad was right, and his confidence enabled me to take another step toward becoming an ordinary person just like everyone else. From that point on, I was able to drive myself to school.

High school flew by, and I was delighted to graduate with the same class I had started school with in the first grade. There was never any question about my going to college after graduation; it was simply expected of me. So I sent for brochures and catalogs from Scripps College in Claremont, California. This school was near my sister's home, and I thought it would be great to live near her.

Mother and I made a trip out to California to see the college. It was a beautiful campus with beautiful buildings, but there was one problem: there were far too many steps. That was an important consideration because steps always posed a big problem for me. I was very disappointed and would have loved to enroll there, but I knew it was necessary to find a school that had no steps. So the search continued.

# *Chapter 5*

*M*ary Jo had attended St. Mary College in Leavenworth, Kansas, so I decided to check it out. This four-year all-girls college was a natural preserve set on 240 acres of rolling hills. As we drove up the long, winding road and entered through the main gate with the name *St. Mary College* emblazoned on it, I was filled with anticipation. It was an absolutely beautiful campus and had a large pond surrounded by trees that led up to the main hall. I loved the peaceful and tranquil atmosphere. And much to my great delight and relief, the campus itself was flat. There was only one building that might pose a problem for me, and it had only three steps. I believed I could find someone to help me with those.

My first year at St. Mary, I shared a suite with three other girls: Joni was my roommate, and Mary Kay and Colleen were my other two suite mates. Keep in mind that I was attending a very traditional, strict Catholic college for girls. Each night, lights out was at ten o'clock, but like most other young women our age, my suite mates and I would often stay awake whispering when we were supposed to be asleep. But we had a surefire method of avoiding detection. As the nun on duty walked in the halls, we could hear the rustle of her rosary beads, and this would alert us to scurry back to bed and pretend to be asleep.

Another restriction we had was that we were not allowed to go into town during the week, only on weekends. But during my senior year, some of the girls sneaked out through a window one night and went into town. Because of my physical limitations, I wasn't able to go with them, which proved to be a blessing in disguise. Needless to say, the girls who participated in this prank were caught, and as a result, half of the class was on restriction and had to sign in every hour for about a month.

Because of the inclement winter weather, the campus had constructed underground tunnels between all the buildings. This setup was perfect for me because now I didn't have to brave the ice and snow. There was also a tunnel leading to the Annunciation Chapel where we attended Mass. In those days, we were required to wear black caps and gowns to Mass, but it really wasn't an inconvenience. In fact, if we overslept, we could simply throw on our gowns over our pajamas and rush to church, and no one was the wiser for it!

Like all the other students, I needed to decide upon a major. I actually wanted to be a dietician, but the sisters at the school would not hear of it. In all fairness to them, they were only looking out for me and feared my physical disabilities would get in the way of achieving that goal. Since I was not able to use my left hand at all, and my right hand was weak from the polio, they were afraid I would burn myself. I accepted their decision.

Next I decided to major in art. This, too, proved to be a problem because all the art classes were held on the second floor of Miege Hall. Remember, this was an all-girls school, so there were no young men to carry me. I then thought about majoring in education and becoming a teacher, but this was not a realistic goal in the fifties, as schools did not hire teachers with disabilities. Finally I decided to major in English literature because the classes were all held on the first floor. Such was my decision-making process in choosing a major!

The first two years of school seemed to fly by. During my junior year, my dad called one day with wonderfully exciting news that would open up new horizons to me that I had never before dreamed of.

# Chapter 6

"*H*ello, Margy. How's everything going?" My Dad greeted me as I answered the phone. We chatted for a while, just talking about usual, ordinary things before he revealed his real reason for calling.

"You know, Margy, I was wondering . . . do you think you would like to go to Europe this summer? I mean, is that something you think you're up to?"

I was taken completely by surprise. "Sure, Daddy, I can do it. I know I can do it! Or if I can't, I'll die trying!"

We both laughed at my overly dramatic remark, but it was settled: I was going to Europe! The college in my hometown was sponsoring a group for a ten-week trip to nine countries, and we would be part of that group.

The rest of the school year flew by, and it was soon time for the long-awaited trip. My mom, dad, a friend of mine named Judy, and I drove to New York and joined the group from the college. We set sail for Europe on the *Johan Van Oldenbarnevelt* (called the *JVO* for short) in Hoboken, New Jersey. It was a glorious departure. We threw colored streamers from the ship's rail and waved to the crowd below, though we didn't know a single person on the dock.

The impressive New York skyline came into view as we glided down the Hudson River, and as we headed out to the open sea, we passed the awe-inspiring view of the Statue of Liberty. Then, as now, I felt privileged to be an American, and seeing this majestic statue in this setting was absolutely breathtaking. I am not ashamed to say the emotion that welled up inside of me was almost overwhelming. We were off to a magnificent start for a magnificent journey.

Though nothing could dampen our unabashed enthusiasm for our great adventure, the *JVO,* in reality, was a twenty-eight-year-old clunker. Mostly college students were aboard. Our cabin was very small, with metal bunks on the right and a drop-down bed in the wall on the left. When the bed frame was lowered, there was barely enough room to squeeze by. As might be expected, my mom was not too happy with the sleeping arrangements, but they were standard accommodations for the college package.

Nothing could dim my excitement, however, and I had a blast with the other students. Every evening we gathered to play cards, listen to music, and take advantage of the eighteen-cent drinks from the bar. My dad couldn't fathom why anyone would want to stay up all night and then sleep all day. But I was having the time of my life, with the added bonus of earning six credits toward my college degree.

On the trip over, my mother and I were eating breakfast one day when we heard a terrible grinding noise. Running to the porthole, we could see nothing that would indicate what had happened. But soon the captain's voice came over the loudspeaker, and he explained that one of the propellers had stopped working. Since we were already halfway to Europe, we would continue our journey with the use of only one propeller. Of course, this slowed our pace considerably—to eight knots an hour—but it was unavoidable. While we were chugging along, we even saw another ship, the *QE2,* cross the ocean, return, and cross again before we ever made land for the first time!

Ten days after leaving Hoboken, we finally arrived in Europe. Passing through the Oranje Lock in the Netherlands, we peered over the rail of the ship to the sight of children wearing wooden shoes. I had always thought this was a fairy tale representation of the Dutch people, but here I was, seeing it with my very own eyes. It was as if my children's picture books of windmills and wooden shoes had burst into life before me.

We soon found our hotel and dropped off our luggage before embarking on yet another boat to travel the canals of Amsterdam. More water! We had just come from almost two weeks at sea, and there we were, on the water again!

Since most of my family were florists, we of course went to see the beautiful flowers at Alsmeer.

Alsmeer, a small town near Amsterdam, boasted acres and acres of blooming flowers. Large fields of brilliant red flowers abutted huge blocks of gorgeous yellow, pink, and lavender flowers. In the middle of this sea of color stood an auction house, where the flowers were auctioned off to international buyers. The auction house was huge, about the size of nine football fields under one roof, and carts of plant material were hooked together and pulled through the auction area. I watched intently as cart after cart of flowers was auctioned off in the rapid-fire speech of the auctioneers. The flowers were immediately shipped and would appear in flower shops all over the world the next morning. It was an incredible experience.

There were so many wonderful things to see, but going to the Rijksmuseum to view the *Night Watch* by Rembrandt is indelibly impressed upon my memory. The colossal painting, measuring twelve by fourteen feet, was displayed in a small dark room and spotlighted very subtly. As I walked into the room, it took my breath away, so absolutely astounding was its greatness. Like the thousands before me who have been privileged to view this masterpiece, my eyes were immediately drawn to the brightness of the two militiamen and the young girl in the painting. Slowly, almost like magic, the shadowy men in the background emerged and came into focus. So spectacular was the effect that I felt like I was actually seeing real people.

After the visit to the Rijksmuseum, we were on the water again as we traveled down the Rhine River. Still standing after World War II, the great cathedral in Cologne was, nevertheless, missing huge sections. Although it had been spared from most of the bombing, the stone walls at ground level were pock-marked from bullets and shells. Viewing the burned-out cavities of churches and buildings, the aftermath of that terrible war, I couldn't even begin to fathom how the people of Europe had endured such devastation. A new appreciation for what America had been spared and the hope that it would always be so welled up within my heart.

After traveling by water for so long, our itinerary shifted, and we began to travel by bus. I was overjoyed, although the new mode of transportation did present some challenges. In order to board the bus, I had to first maneuver the steps. My dad and I worked out a method, though, that actually worked pretty well. For each step, I would first place my right (good) leg on a step, and then my dad would lift up my brace leg. We repeated the procedure for each step until I was finally aboard the bus. Getting off the bus wasn't nearly as difficult. In order to see all the sights, I had to do this several times a time, but I didn't complain. I was in Europe and having the time of my life!

Traveling by bus, we soon arrived at Lake Constance in Austria. Bordered by three countries, Lake Constance occupies an extremely beautiful corner of central Europe. Near the lake was a small village named St. Anton. Nestled at the foot of the picturesque Alps, the village was too small to have any hotels, so we roomed at a private home. In the morning, surrounded by the awesome snowcapped

Alps, we ate a leisurely breakfast on the porch of the quaint little house.

Later that day as my mother and I were enjoying lunch in a café in town, we were gazing out the window and noticed a procession traveling up the road in our direction. As the procession came into view, we saw an ox pulling a cart with a casket on top. A priest and a few people were following behind, saying the rosary.

As we watched the little group wind its way along the road, suddenly, much to our astonishment, we recognized a familiar face: My dad! *What in the world?* . . . I thought, and I glanced at Mom, who seemed to be thinking the exact same thing. Later we discovered that when my dad had seen the procession with the people saying the rosary, he had decided to pray with them. He even went all the way to the grave site, throwing dirt onto the grave and then speaking to the priest.

Daddy was told that the person in the casket was a young man who had been killed in a skiing accident. Even more tragic, this young man had escaped through the iron curtain from East Germany to Austria. With his family still in East Germany, there was no money for a proper funeral. My kind-hearted father, upon hearing the sad story, immediately gave the priest enough money to cover the funeral expenses and to have masses said for the young man for the next five years. When we returned to Missouri, a letter from his parents had arrived, thanking my father for his kindness. (Of course, it was written in German, and we couldn't understand it; so we took it to the college to have it translated.) But the entire experience only reinforced what I already knew about my dad: he was a kind, generous man, always thinking of others and willing to share with those in need.

In Venice, Italy, we took to the water again as we traversed the famous canals of the old city. By this time, I was getting pretty good at maneuvering into boats and not falling into the water; nevertheless, the rocking, swaying gondolas did pose a challenge. Once again, I managed, learning all the while that polio did not have to be a debilitating handicap. For the most part, I could always find a way to do what I really wanted to do.

That's not to say that there weren't some moments when my physical limitations did present some very unique—even comical—situations. In Venice, we stayed in a very charming but older hotel with a communal bathroom down the hall. To lock the door, you had to use a heavy, old-fashioned key. I managed to lock the door just fine, but when I was ready to get out, I couldn't turn the key because of the trouble I have with my hands. I was locked inside!

At the time, it didn't seem all that humorous, but in retrospect, there was quite an element of comedy to it. There I was, alone and helplessly locked in the bathroom, while my parents, the bellboy, and the manager on the other side of the door were all loudly and excitedly trying to figure out a way to rescue me.

"Margy . . . Margy . . . stay calm," came my mother's reassuring voice over the agitated exclamations of the men. "We'll have you out in a minute."

"I'm okay, Mom. I'm fine, really," I answered. And I was fine. I knew I couldn't stay locked in there forever. I knew my dad or one of the others would eventually figure something out.

"Margy," now my father spoke, "the bellboy is going to shimmy through the transom at the top. Then he can unlock the door for you. We'll have you out in no time." It seemed everyone was trying to reassure me, but I think maybe they were trying to reassure themselves!

As planned, the bellboy got a ladder to reach the transom, but he couldn't fit through the opening. It was too small, so that plan didn't work.

A light bulb seemed to pop on in my mind. "Hey . . . everyone . . . I know what we can do. I'll throw the key out the window, and then you can retrieve it and unlock the door from your side." Murmurs of agreement came from the other side of the door, and plan two was launched. In no time, I was free, and later we all laughingly remarked how fortunate we were that the window had not faced the canal side of the street!

Next stop: Rome! Here in the ancient city I experienced one of the most memorable and spiritually uplifting experiences of the trip. My dad met a woman who was the superintendent of Catholic schools in New York City. She had passes to go to the Vatican to see the pope and asked if we were going. Although we had indeed planned to do so, we hadn't known we needed passes, so the woman was kind enough to add our names to her list.

Arriving at St. Peter's Basilica, my dad was helping me up the steps of the church when a member from the Swiss Guards approached and offered a wheelchair. Although we didn't understand his words, we understood his intention as he motioned for me to sit in the chair. This I was happy to do. No sooner had I seated myself than the guard whisked me away up the right side of the church. He was a very tall man, and my shorter dad had to literally run alongside to keep up with the guard's long strides.

St. Peter's is huge, several football fields in length and width, and there is much to see in this sacred site. The *Pietà* by Michelangelo is located in the first chapel to the right, and as we passed it, we saw people leaning over to kiss the base of the statue. So many people over so many years have expressed their reverence for this depiction of Jesus resting on his mother's lap after His crucifixion that a large worn spot has developed.

That mark, however, is a mark of piety and reverence, unlike the tragic vandalism directed against the masterpiece on Pentecost Sunday in 1972. On that day, a mentally disturbed geologist walked into the chapel and attacked the Virgin with a geologist's hammer while shouting, "I am Jesus Christ!" The *Pietà* has since been restored and is now protected by a bulletproof acrylic glass panel. Such are the days we live in, but none of that marred my day in the Vatican that summer.

The guard wheeled me past the *Pietà* to the front of the papal altar located next to a double ramp of stairs. The basilica centers around this papal altar, where only the pope celebrates Mass. Rising above the altar is the baldacchino, a magnificent ninety-five-foot canopy. The stairs from the basilica descend into a semicircle leading to the tomb of St. Peter, which is under the altar. The area there is beautifully illuminated by the eternal flames of one hundred lamps.

While we were waiting for the pope to arrive, I had an interesting conversation with a lady standing next to me. She looked at me for a moment before inquiring, "If you don't mind my asking, why are you in that wheelchair?"

"Well, six years ago I contracted polio," I explained. "I can walk with the help of a leg brace and crutches, but sometimes it's easier and more practical to use the wheelchair."

The woman nodded her head thoughtfully before answering, "My daughter, Mary, had polio too, when she was nineteen, but unfortunately, she did not survive."

I sat quietly, sympathizing with her, when she interrupted my thoughts with, "Oh, let me introduce myself. I'm Helen Hayes, and this is my son James."

Helen Hayes! There I sat, chatting with the "first lady of Broadway" and her son, James MacArthur, later of *Hawaii Five-O* television fame. Before I could think of how I should answer, our conversation was interrupted by a commotion at the door of the basilica. Pope Pius XII was being carried in on a sedan chair on the shoulders of the Swiss Guards. People were shouting, "''Vive il Papa!''. . . ''Vive il Papa!''. . .," or "Long live the pope!" The guards lowered the chair, and the pope got off and started reaching out his hands to touch and bless people. Some people especially wanted their babies to receive a blessing, so they passed their children through the crowd in order to reach the pope. We are all quite excited and awestruck with this holy man in our midst.

Suddenly Pope Pius was right there in front of me. Gently placing his hand upon my head, he gave me his blessing. As I was kissing his ring, as was customary, I heard him kindly inquire of my father, "What is wrong with your daughter, sir?"

We were devout Catholics, and my father, overwhelmed by the pope's proximity and kindness, could barely speak. In a broken voice, he managed to get out, "Your Holiness, it's polio."

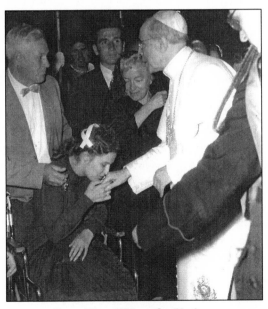

**Pope Pius XII at the Vatican**

Pope Pius simply looked at me and smiled, and as I met his gaze, I looked into the most beautiful blue eyes in the world. There was a surreal depth to them, as though the owner of these gentle eyes could not possibly belong to this world. The pope continued making his way through the crowd, speaking and blessing as he went. When he passed me again, he blessed me a second time. Then he climbed the steps to the altar and spoke to the crowd in several different languages.

This day, July 23, 1958, was not only a memorable day for me and my family but also for all Catholics. Though unknown at the time, that day was Pius XII's last public audience. He died eleven weeks later on October 9 at his summer home, Castel Gandolfo. Over forty years later, in the year 2000, Pope John Paul II bestowed the title of "Venerable" upon Pope Pius XII, which is the last step before a person is canonized as a saint in the Roman Catholic Church. Just think—one day I may be able to say that I was blessed by a saint!

As we were leaving after this exhilarating experience, a nun approached us and asked if we realized that the Associated Press had taken our picture. We had not been aware of that, but of course we wanted copies. The nun told us where we could pick up the pictures, but we were leaving that afternoon for Nice and would not be able to get them. Seeing our dilemma, she kindly offered to retrieve the pictures and mail them to us, which she did. When my dad died a number of years later, we discovered that he had been sending money to the orphanage she headed for the previous ten years before his death. That was the kind of man he was: quietly doing right, always going beyond the call of duty, motivated by the generosity and love that the heavenly Father had planted in his heart.

Breathtaking landscapes, interesting cultural outings, and deep spiritual experiences were not the only things that occupied my time, though. In an art gallery in Italy, I met a young, good-looking guy named Checcio Menio from the town of Genore. We talked for quite some time and hit it off so well that the next day he decided to board the train to Monte Carlo, where my family and I were headed. The perfect gentleman, Checcio carried my suitcases, assisted me up the steps onto the train, and bought us a glass of wine from the porter.

Many of the other passengers also bought wine, and before long we were all literally hanging out the open windows of the train. Needless to say, we were enjoying ourselves immensely and even growing quite boisterous, especially when the train speeded around a curve. Much to our delight and humor, we could look out our window and see the people in the car behind us coming around the curve as they watched us exit the curve. We gleefully shouted and waved to one another, and by the time we arrived in Monte Carlo, we were all great buddies.

After I returned home, my Italian sweetheart wrote to me for many months. He couldn't write English, so his friend wrote the letters for him. That did not deter him, however, from writing some really great love letters!

In Barcelona, Spain, we stayed in a beautiful hotel. After arriving and depositing our luggage at the hotel, we immediately departed for a bullfight. The bullfight was held outside in an arena with concrete bleachers that had enormously high steps. Struggling to climb the steps, I fell and got a bad cut, so I was forced to leave and find first aid. I didn't mind, though; I was really put off with the whole obscene idea of killing a bull under the guise of "entertainment."

After the bullfight, we all piled into a taxi for the ride back to the hotel, but we soon realized we had a problem: no one could remember the name of the hotel where we were staying! We drove around for hours looking for it. We saw a policeman directing traffic and began trying to describe the hotel to him, with hopes that he would be able to point us in the right direction. Unfortunately, the only thing we could remember was that it was on a corner. Obviously, that was not much help. Finally, through trial and error more than anything else, we found our hotel and went in for a much needed rest.

Later that day, my mom, Judy, and I decided to go shopping. My mother was pushing my wheelchair when the tires got snagged on the streetcar tracks. Before she could free me, however, a streetcar came into view, clanging and clanging for me to get out of the way. Everyone was frantically waving and yelling in Spanish for me to move. I wasn't really all that afraid of the streetcar as much as I was of all the wildly excitable people. Some men came to the rescue and pried my chair free and placed me back on the curb, out of harm's way.

It seemed that everywhere we went, I faced one type of challenge or another, some more difficult than others. One rather embarassing moment occurred in a little town in the Pyrenees Mountains. The main street of this quaint village was so narrow that it could not accommodate two vehicles at once. When a car approached our bus from the opposite direction, our driver was forced to drive partially on the sidewalk to make allowance for the other vehicle.

We laughed about that, giving it little thought, but when we made a bathroom stop, our laughter soon changed to dismay. The ladies' "bathroom" consisted of a room with a concrete floor with a drain in the middle. Footprints marked either side of the drain. Startled at the crude accommodations, I couldn't imagine how I was going to manage something as simple as going to the bathroom. Fortunately, the women from the bus helped my mother hold me over the drain. Embarrassing, yes—but I was oh so grateful!

Lourdes, in the southwestern part of France, was our next stop. This is the site of the apparitions of Our Lady of Lourdes in 1858 to Bernadette Soubirous, a fourteen-year- old peasant girl. One day as Bernadette was gathering firewood with her sister and a friend, the Lady first appeared to her. Subsequent appearances followed, and on one of these occasions, Bernadette was instructed to drink from the water at the site. As Bernadette obeyed, the muddy water became increasingly clear. As the word of this miracle spread, the healing water was given to many sick people, and many miraculous cures were reported, either from drinking the water or bathing in it. One Easter Sunday, the Lady identified herself to Bernadette with, "I am the Immaculate Conception." Bernadette was beatified in 1925 and canonized in 1933.

After arriving at Lourdes, I went to the Grotto. The water from the springs there is believed to possess healing properties, and the Roman Catholic Church officially recognizes occasional miraculous healings. At the site, a "ministry of welcome" for both males and females receive the sick and the infirm. The women at the springs helped me disrobe and then wrapped a sheet around me. Into the icy healing water I went, and teeth chattering, I made my way to the statue of the Virgin at the other end and sat down in the water for about a minute. Miraculous Cave, or the Cave of Apparitions, is a large recessed area with an altar, and when I looked into it, I imagined Our Lady standing there. In front of the grotto was a large candle holder with many candles placed there by countless worshipers.

During the fifteenth apparition, Our Lady had given a special message to Bernadette. "Go tell the priests to come here in procession and to build a chapel here," she instructed. Her words were obeyed, and that afternoon I was part of the "procession of the sick." As we lined up in three rows, the bishop passed by and blessed us with the Blessed Sacrament. I was not physically healed at Lourdes, but the spiritual impact was great, nonetheless.

Interlaken, Switzerland, whose name literally means "between two lakes," sported an aerial car that ascended to four thousand feet. The idyllic view overlooking the lush green valley with the sparkling lakes and snowcapped mountains was nothing short of breathtaking. But in order to take advantage of the spectacular view, we had to board a gondola, an enclosed structure suspended from a cable. At first I had no reservations about the ride, although the gondola was making ominous creaking noises. But as I sat on a bench and gazed out the window, the slowly receding land suddenly melted away with a drop that seemed to make the land below a million miles away. A house down below now looked like nothing more than a miniature doll house.

I was petrified and didn't want to move, as though that could in some way ensure my protection. Frozen with fear, I clutched the side of my seat until we finally reached the opposite side. I couldn't wait to disembark and escape from the aerial prison. But of course I had to ride the gondola back down the mountain, and after we ate lunch in the restaurant, it was time to start the dreaded return.

Most of my life, I have gone with the flow, rarely bucking the current or causing a scene. Partly, I suppose, that is my nature, and partly, that is the way I was raised. But all that flew out the window now, so deep was my fear. I simply refused to get back into the gondola, certain that death awaited me if I did.

"Margy, be reasonable. We've got to go back, and you've got to ride the gondola. Come on, honey.

It'll be all right," Mom said in the most reassuring voice she could muster.

But when fear takes root, common sense flies out the window, and that's where I was. "Please, don't make me ride in that thing. It'll crash; I just know it will. Isn't there another way down the mountain? There's got to be another way. I can't ride in that thing—I just can't." I was so scared by this point that I actually began to cry. But there was little my parents could do—there was no other way back but by gondola.

Somehow they finally persuaded me to board, but I was so frightened I could do nothing more than huddle in a corner, close my eyes, and pray we would all make it to safety. The trip back seemed to take forever. I was on full alert, listening for the first hint of trouble that would tell me that the cable was about to break and send us all down to certain death. I was so badly shaken by the entire episode that when we later visited Zurich, Bern, and Geneva, I limited myself to what I could view from the solid ground— not from a flimsy gondola dangling on a cable!

Vive la Paris—the city of love! Paris fairly pulsated with excitement and energy. Blaring horns and the lyrical sounds of the French language exuded a vibrancy unmatched by any city we had previously visited. The drivers in Paris, particularly the taxi drivers, careened at breakneck speed through the city streets as though they were driving on a racetrack. You took your life in your hands when crossing a street, and I had to be particularly careful since I couldn't move fast.

Having taken a French class in college, I was already aware of all the fascinating sites of the city, places like the Eiffel Tower, Versailles, and the Hall of Mirrors, and looked forward to seeing them. But one place I had never learned about in my all-girls college was Pigalle.

Pigalle, located in the old red-light district of Paris, is a popular tourist attraction and a curious blend of beautiful landmark burlesque theaters mixed with very bourgeois buildings. Our group decided to venture to the Pigalle to see the famous Apache dancers' performance in a club there. The Apache dance originated in the Parisian lower classes at the beginning of the twentieth century and is a sort of "over the top" tango.

We watched mesmerized as the male dancer, as part of his routine, would throw the female dancer across the floor; the rejected woman would pick herself up and go back to him, clinging to him as he strutted away. During one part of the dance, the male dancer strutted over to our table and proceeded to sit on my lap, much to my surprise. The woman jerked him off and grabbed my neck and shook it as if she were choking me. It was all part of the act, but not liking to be in the spotlight, I was embarrassed by all the attention. The audience, on the other hand, thought it was tremendously funny.

The most interesting place in Paris was the Louvre. In 1958 a person could actually walk up and touch the *Mona Lisa*. Aspiring artists positioned their easels in the vicinity and gathered around to try their skill at painting the timeless beauty.

An impressive sight in the Esplanade des Invalides was the mahogany tomb of Napoleon. Done on a gargantuan scale, the tomb sits in the center of a vast opening. There is an eight-foot statue of the emperor in his coronation robes, and the tomb itself is located on the floor beneath where visitors stand. To view the tomb, a person has to lean over a rail to look down at it. It is said that Napoleon left specific instructions for his tomb to be built in just this way so that everyone who came to see it would, in effect, have to bow before him.

After an unforgettable time in Paris, we headed for Brussels, Belgium. We were traveling by train, but my group was running late and was last to board. We cut it rather close, however. I remember having my right foot on the bottom step and my left one poised in the air as the train began to move. The porter was holding one of my arms and my dad the other as they tugged me aboard. I remember looking down and observing that the ground was moving, though of course it wasn't really the ground but the train that was moving.

Brussels was an exciting destination because it was the site of the first world's fair to be held since World War II. So immense was the location that we immediately got separated from our group. However, we quickly hired one of the motorcycle carts available for transport and began our search for them. I had never ridden on a motorcycle before, but I climbed into the cart with my dad and held on to him and the driver as we fairly flew around the fairgrounds. We didn't find our group, but we did get a quick overview of the fair.

The United States' pavilion was quite a popular attraction. It was composed of a large round building with a lake and lots of waterfalls in front as well as small models of American homes featuring all the newest appliances and gadgets. It also spotlighted the American drugstore, which became the highlight of the entire fair. The drugstore sold milkshakes, sundaes, and fifty-cent Cokes, which was quite expensive in those days. In fact, only the rich could afford the Cokes, and I was reminded again of the abundance that we Americans often take for granted. But even more popular than the Cokes was the great American dessert: ice cream! Everyone was quite enraptured with the ice cream, so much so that long lines snaked around as people waited their turns to enter the drugstore.

Unsuccessul at finding our group, we decided to head back to the entrance but soon discovered we had a problem: there were eleven entrances! We had left my wheelchair at one of them, so we had to frantically race around trying to find it, which we eventually did. We were on a tight schedule, but we managed to make it to the boat train and depart for England, our next stop.

Daddy, however, stayed behind in Belgium for a couple of days, a time I labeled as his "lost weekend." Later when he caught up with us in England, he explained that he had stayed behind to visit his family's place of origin: Renaix, Belgium. His grandfather and my great-grandfather, Vital DeBacker, had worked as a miller at his father's windmill prior to leaving Belgium for Kansas in 1883. Flipping through the phone book, Dad found page after page of DeBacker's listed, much to his amazement. Back home, we were the only DeBacker's we had ever heard of. Even more amazing was the fact that he saw a flower shop with the sign "DeBacker," hanging over the door, and as I've already mentioned, my family owned DeBacker's Flower Shop in Warrensburg, Missouri.

It was thrilling to learn this part of my family's history and later when my daughter was born, I named her Renée, pronounced "ren-NAY," just like the Flemish town of my ancestors.

The thirty-cent boat-train ride across the English Channel was an event! The tiny boat was crammed full, and the waves were fierce and choppy. On top of that, a few of the passengers were unpleasantly seasick. Because of the conditions, no one was allowed on the deck. We all had to go below, and the only way down was by way of a ladder. Sitting on the floor, I scooted over to the opening; then two men lifted me down by my shoulders.

There were about twenty people crowded into this small area, and there were no chairs and only a few bunks. The boat was rocking quite a bit, and I was having trouble standing, so Mom began asking if someone would give up their bunk for me. No one wanted to, but Mom kept insisting. Although no one spoke English, she made her request known and persisted until one lady was kind enough to relinquish her bunk for me. Mom, however, was forced to stand for the entire crossing, and, like the other passengers, was tossed about tremendously. Thankfully, it wasn't long before we docked in Dover, England. The white cliffs of Dover—I had read about them, and now I was actually seeing them! What a sight!

On the train to London, we relished a tasty breakfast of eggs and toast instead of the usual hard rolls and coffee we had eaten for the past two months. It was a welcome change of fare. While in London, we stayed busy visiting the usual attractions, but one day I stayed behind alone in my room while the rest of the group went sightseeing. However, I soon changed my mind, thinking it rather silly to sit in a hotel room when I could be seeing the sights in London. Though somewhat apprehensive about going anywhere by myself, I thought, *I have money. I'll just hire a cab and ride around and see things.* The hotel called a taxi for me, and I directed the driver to park across the street from Buckingham Palace where I could watch the changing of the guard. I was quite pleased with figuring out a way to go out on my own!

We left Southampton, England, for the trip home aboard the German *Hanseatic.* Unlike our crossing at the beginning of the journey, this time we had a beautiful and very large suite. Instead of a small cabin with metal beds, we enjoyed the luxury of a queen-sized bed, a sofa, a chair, and a round table within our suite.

The weather was as good as it possibly could be in the North Atlantic, and we were making good time until we hit the tail end of a hurricane. Being young and rather ignorant about hurricanes, I wasn't afraid at all of the rough seas, but rather quite exhilarated by the entire experience. The ship tossed back and forth, and when I made my way along the corridors, I could go only a few feet at a time. Mom and I walked arm in arm and zigzagged from place to place as the wind continued to blow and the sea continued to churn. Eventually the wind and rough seas subsided, and we arrived home from our glorious European adventure.

# *Chapter 7*

*H*ome from my travels, I soon got back into the groove of school, and my last year of college was over in the blink of an eye. It was an exciting day when final exams were finally over: no more metaphysics, no more logic classes, and no more trying to understand books like *The Essence of Knowledge*. I knew I wouldn't miss my classes one bit, but I would miss my classmates.

Like all graduations, it was a bittersweet time. I was sad to be leaving behind all the wonderful memories and friendships of my college days, but at the same time, the future beckoned brightly. The big day finally arrived, and the graduation ceremony was held outside at Xavier Hall. Each girl was to walk up the steps to be handed her diploma by the college president, but in my case, the president graciously walked down to me and awarded me that all-important paper that said I'd earned a bachelor's degree in English.

Now it was time to find a job. I had a college degree in hand and thought that should open doors for me. And though I was right about that in many respects, what I had not taken into account was the fact that my physical disabilities closed some of the very doors my diploma opened. I discovered this the hard way when I went to Arizona to apply for an opening at an AAA travel agency. After the interview, I looked for an apartment, but every apartment I found had at least one step. Unable to manage even one step on my own, I realized I was not going to be able to live alone. This was a crushing blow! Not knowing what else to do, I resigned myself to the fact that I would have to get a job in Warrensburg and live with my parents.

Returning home, I applied and was hired as a receptionist at the Warrensburg Medical Center, making sixty-five cents an hour. I was receptionist for both the hospital and seven doctors with offices in the same building. Although it was very busy and loads of fun, and I did meet lots of interesting people while answering phones and signing patients in, I certainly wasn't using my bachelor's degree. But sometimes things work out in unexpected ways, and that's what happened in my new job.

A few months after I started working at the hospital, a friend invited me to double date with her and her boyfriend. I consented to the setup and went out that night with Bob Dieguez, a young airman from Whiteman, the nearby air force base. On our first date, we went to a drive-in movie and had a wonderful time.

We continued seeing each other, and soon we became inseparable. Every chance he had, Bob picked me up at the hospital to take me to lunch. At night he would take me to the movies or to a play at the local college. Our relationship was progressing quickly.

Then one night after we had gone to a play, Bob was not acting like himself. It seemed like he had something on his mind. He was nervous and jittery, and instead of starting up the car when we got in, he just sat there, very still.

*What's up with Bob?* I wondered. *He sure doesn't seem like himself. I wonder if I did something to upset him.* My thoughts were suddenly interrupted when Bob, unceremoniously and without warning, blurted out, "Margy, will you marry me?"

Astounded, I sat there for just a moment before giving him an emphatic yes. Then he reached across to the glove compartment, took out a small box, and gave me a beautiful diamond ring.

Of course, we went home to tell my parents our big news, but my parents were not at all happy about it. Later my dad and our parish priest tried to talk me out of the marriage, but I was starry-eyed and stubborn and wouldn't listen to either of them. A year after we had met, Bob and I married. I wore the beautiful mantilla my parents bought in Florence, Italy for my brother's new wife, Franny. On the big day, I was thrilled to walk down the aisle on my dad's arm without even using my crutches.

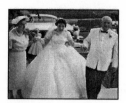

***Get me to the church on time***

I soon settled into the routine of being a new wife and setting up my first home. When I worked at the hospital, I had been able to save a little money because I lived with my parents and didn't have any living expenses. So Bob and I used that to buy a little forty-by-eight-foot trailer. Small as it was, I thought it was wonderful. I had my very own place with my very own husband! But I did have to make some adjustments to accommodate my physical reality.

Because of the weakness in my hands, I had not been allowed to take cooking classes in college, but now I would be cooking for a husband in my own kitchen. I hadn't cooked at all since contracting polio at fifteen, so I had a lot to learn and needed to think of different ways to do everyday jobs. For instance, peeling potatoes with a knife was out of the question, so I boiled them with the skins on and then peeled them. When I carried a saucepan from the sink to the stove, I would use my left wrist to stabilize the pan while gripping it with my right hand. I had to be very careful to make sure that the contents weren't too heavy. But I was a fast learner, and whatever problems I encountered, I set to work to find a way to solve them.

Then it happened: I got pregnant. Lo and behold, everyone was so upset! Everyone wondered how I would be able to take care of a baby, and their concern was somewhat justified, considering I had never even held a baby. But that was obviously a moot point now, and I would have to figure out a way to care for my child, just as I had figured out a way to cook for my husband.

Up until the last month, my pregnancy was wonderfully uneventful. But in that last month, my blood pressure shot up to over two hundred and wouldn't come down. Also, my body was terribly swollen and as big as a beach ball; I felt like someone had inserted a hose into me and puffed me up like a balloon. I was admitted into the hospital, doctor's orders.

My condition was diagnosed: preeclampsia, a life-threatening condition. The doctor was monitoring me carefully and soon decided I needed an emergency caesarean section. Informing my husband and parents that he might not be able to save the baby, the doctor promised he would try his best to at least save me. Thankfully, he saved us both. My baby boy, Robby, was born healthy, and my life, too, was spared; but I was too sick to be aware of anything for a while. For the first three days following Robby's birth, the nurses regularly brought him to me, but I wasn't even able to hold him. When I became more alert, the doctor advised me against having any more children, warning that I might not survive the next time. I was crushed because I very much wanted to have another child.

Robby was so little, just six pounds. His little bottom was so small I had to use handkerchiefs for diapers. Before he was born, I had tried to think of a way to diaper him. Disposable diapers had not yet made their appearance, so I had to figure out a way to fasten Robby's cloth diapers. I came up with the idea of using Velcro in place of pins; however, that method didn't work for long because the baby soon outgrew the placement of the Velcro tabs. So I devised another method by pulling the back side of the diaper to the front, folding it to make it thick, and then laying a thin piece of the cloth from the front on top. I steadied all of this with my left wrist and then ran a large baby pin through both pieces. It worked, and Robby did not get stuck even once.

Carrying the baby from one room to another proved to be more difficult, but I found a way to make it work. When I wanted to pick Robby up, I would lean over his baby bed, scoot him to my left arm, and then pull him to my chest. Once he was in my arms, I would walk beside the walls to steady myself without my crutches. Soon I didn't even need the wall anymore.

As Robby grew older, he would put his little arms around my neck when I leaned over his bed so that I could lift and carry him when I straightened up. After he learned to crawl, I placed a box in front of the couch and another in front of his high chair so he could climb up when necessary. Robby accepted my unique style of mothering with no complaint. My mother insisted he knew not to wiggle when I changed his diaper or to run away from me. I don't know if that was true, but we did learn to adapt to each other just like any mother and child.

In my spare time, I began making ceramic nativities, carolers, and lots of flower vases, which my parents used for flower arrangements at their flower shop. The ceramics were fired in my kiln, and I had one large room to hold my molds, paints, and other necessary materials. It was difficult to keep my hand steady while doing the detail work, such as with the doll faces, but I managed. Making and painting ceramics became a small business and a way to add a little to our income.

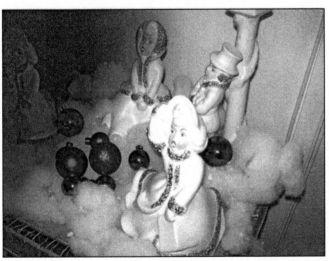

*Christmas carolers*

My husband lost his job in Kansas City, so we decided to move to California. Bob got a job with Sears, and I was hired at a private Catholic school in Tujunga. My college teachers had discouraged me from going into education, saying no one would hire me as a teacher, but I was hired and successfully taught fifty-two third-graders. What a challenge! Walking around in the classroom, I wore my leg brace, and I was now able to walk without crutches most of the time.

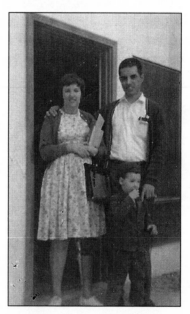

***Off to a day of teaching***

Well, time passed, and I did what my doctor told me not to do: I got pregnant again. Realizing that this was a high-risk pregnancy, I went to UCLA Medical Center because I had heard that it was a very good hospital. I knew that if anyone could get me through this pregnancy, they could.

Much as it had been with my first pregnancy, everything was fine at first, but in the last three months, my blood pressure started to spike again. I was ordered on total bed rest and given phenobarbital to keep me quiet and rested. It was a difficult time because my husband was working and my little three-year-old boy needed care and attention. Robby would play quietly in the fenced backyard while I rested, and a thoughtful neighbor kept an eye on him for me. Fortunately, I had no problem with the delivery of my little girl, Renee. She was so sweet and tiny, and when she puckered her lips, they looked like a little rosebud.

Despite the joy my children brought, I was having problems with Bob. Many times he would get upset about something and storm out of the house, shouting he was leaving forever. Sometimes he would be gone for an hour, and other times he would be gone for four or five hours. At first his actions frightened me, but as I grew accustomed to his unpredictable behavior, my fear changed to annoyance. Just six weeks after Renee's birth, Bob left and stayed gone for two weeks, the longest he had ever been gone. This time was different, too, because he took the money from our checking and savings accounts and left me alone with a newborn baby to care for.

During those two weeks of Bob's absence, others pitched in to help. Bob's father and mother and my sister brought me food, and the milkman kindly provided my milk for free. When Bob finally returned, he acted as if he had just come back from the drugstore.

"Hi, Margy. How's it going?" he nonchalantly remarked as he cheerfully walked into the house, all smiles. "Where's Robby, and how's the baby?"

I could hardly believe his cavalier attitude. Keeping my emotions firmly reined in, I answered in a tight, short voice. "I'm fine, and so are the kids—if you really care to know. But, you know, Bob, you can't just waltz out of our lives like that and come back when you feel like it and expect everything to be just fine. It doesn't work that way, and I'm not willing to live like that anymore. If you want to make a home with me and the kids, then you've got to agree to marriage counseling. If you can't agree to that, then I think you should leave."

Bob's smile faded from his face, and his entire demeanor changed. But he did agree to go to counseling with me, and it seemed to help. For the next year, things were pretty good between us, and life went on.

I decided to take cake decorating classes and discovered that with practice and patience, I could master the new skill. Like so many other things in my life, I just had to figure out a creative way to do what I wanted to do. To decorate the cakes, I would press the icing bag against my chin and use my one good hand to squeeze out the frosting. In this way, I decorated and sold train cakes, wedding cakes, and holiday cakes. I even made a doll cake for Renee's first birthday.

During this busy time in my life, another unexpected thrill came my way. The TV show *Let's Make a Deal* was recorded in Burbank near where we lived.

This was a popular game show where people dressed up in crazy costumes hoping to be chosen by Monty Hall, the show's host, who would then offer to make them a deal. Bob and I decided to give it a try.

For the show, I made a red flannel nightgown with a red and white striped ruffle at the bottom. Bob donned the nightgown, as well as a red nightcap with a white tassel at the end, and carried a huge white candle for special effect. To our great delight, Bob was selected as a contestant, and Monty Hall offered him a deal: Bob could choose whatever was written on a piece of paper in a certain balloon, or he could have whatever was behind a curtain on stage. Bob chose the balloon.

The curtain opened to reveal seven old Maytag washing machines, and then Monty Hall popped the balloon to see what Bob's prize would be. Inside was a paper that said, "You are going on a trip." Another curtain opened and showed a Pan Am jet, and then yet another curtain opened and showed the Royal Hawaiian Hotel. Known as the Pink Palace of the Pacific, the Royal Hawaiian is a luxurious, exclusive resort on the breathtaking Waikiki beachfront frequented by movie stars and wealthy patrons. Bob had won a week's vacation in Hawaii, plus four hundred dollars spending money! We used the money for a down payment and closing costs on a new house, however, so had to eat at the five-and-dime store while on our luxury vacation!

When we first arrived at our hotel room, an enormous basket of fruit awaited us. In the fifties, we only had canned pineapple available to us in Missouri, so this was my first time to taste fresh pineapple. It was wonderful, like so much of the vacation.

One thing, however, did mar the getaway and was a harbinger of what was looming on the horizon. One particular evening, Bob and I attended a luau at the hotel. After the dinner portion, Bob announced he was going back to the room because he was upset about something, although I did not know what. He left and never returned for me, so I had to ask a bellboy to help me back to the room. Bob was sound asleep, oblivious to anything else, and deep inside I sensed his erratic behavior was starting again.

We returned home and moved into our new home, but things with Bob rapidly deteriorated. Constant chaos and drama ruled our lives, and tension hung thickly in the air. Something as simple as a spilled glass of milk could set Bob off and unleash a torrent of screaming.

Only four months after we had moved into the house, everything came to a head. I was visiting a friend next door when Robby ran up to me, distraught and in tears. "Pops got the car packed, and he said he's leaving forever," my little boy sobbed.

Something snapped in me. Bob had made this threat for the last time, as far as I was concerned. This was it; I'd taken all I could take. It was over! Following up on my new resolve, I called a lock-smith and changed the locks on the door. Later when Bob returned, just as he had so many times before, I held my ground. I could not be dissuaded and firmly insisted, "No more! It's over!" And I meant it.

# *Chapter 8*

*R*ealizing I had to take care of me and my children by myself, I went back to school. I already had my bachelor's degree and one year of teaching experience. The education department at California State University at Northridge (CSUN) believed I would have no problem getting a job if I had my teaching credentials and encouraged me in this new endeavor.

In taking stock of everything, I had a six-year-old boy and a two-year-old baby girl to provide for, car payments and house payments to meet, food to put on the table, and all the responsibilities that come with being a parent. I drove an hour each way for classes, but somehow I found time to take care of my family and keep up with my studies. To help make ends meet, I took a job at the CSUN library, where I worked between classes, and sold Beeline clothes at night and on weekends. If I couldn't find a babysitter, I took my children with me to my Beeline parties.

But even with my part-time work, my income was not adequate, and I was forced to take out a loan.

On my way home from school one day, I stopped at a gas station near my home. A neighbor was there and greeted me rather strangely. Walking up to me, with no preliminaries, she asked, "Have you been home yet?" Her voice sounded worried, and her face reflected the same emotion.

"No . . . I'm on my way there now," I answered slowly. "Why? Is there something wrong?"

"Uh . . . well . . . I was just wondering . . . ," she hurriedly replied as she quickly got into her car and drove off.

Not having a clue as to what was going on, fear gripped my heart as I raced home. *What if something has happened to one of the kids? . . . What if someone has been hurt? . . . Why did she want to know if I had been home yet? . . . Why wouldn't she tell me anything?* The thoughts swirled madly through my head. Finally, I pulled up to my house and saw all my furniture out on the front lawn. *What in the world?* I wondered.

When I left home that day, I had left a lamp on in the living room. I also had a broken window in that room, and the wind had blown through it, knocking over the lamp, which set my curtains on fire. Fortunately, my neighbor had seen the fire and called the fire department. The damage was confined mainly to my living room, although the entire house had suffered smoke damage. But I was just happy that at least my house was still standing and no one had been injured.

During this time of transition and struggle, I was eligible for food stamps, which was a great blessing to me. I never felt ashamed of using them because I knew that it was only temporary and that the assistance enabled me to work toward my independence. But not everyone takes a kind view toward those using food stamps, and I witnessed this firsthand several times.

Once a man behind me in line made the comment, "These people who use food stamps ought to go out and work for a living." He was upset because it took me a while to get the stamps out because of my hands and a little longer for the cashier to process them. Later when I recounted the episode to my mother, she was quite upset and asked me, "Did you show him your hands? That would shut him up"; and Robby, ever the protector, indignantly added, "I wish I was there when they say stuff like that! I'd tell them!"

But I just shrugged it off and thought to myself, *Oh well, too bad!* and went merrily about my business. I knew the truth, and that was all that mattered. I was grateful for any help I received, whether from the school, which paid for my books, or the Encino Women's Club of California, which provided me with some much needed cash. I continued using the food stamps, and when Christmas rolled around, Sierra Vista School generously provided us with a box of food and presents for the kids. I knew I needed help and was thankful for it.

My furnace stopped working the second year we lived in the house. Since I didn't have the money to replace it, I came up with a rather ingenious way to keep the house warm. I bought several pieces of two-by-two sections of wood to make frames for all the windows and then stapled heavy plastic onto the frames. At night I put these handmade storm windows over the regular windows to keep the cold out and then took them off in the morning to let the sun in to warm the house. I also turned the gas stove on for a few minutes each morning to take the chill from the house. It may not have been the best method, but it worked for us.

When my house was built, there had been only two streets with houses, and the surrounding area was nothing but a dense growth of bushes and shrubs. Our house was the last house on our street in this new tract called Timberlane. One year a terrible fire erupted in the hills surrounding our neighborhood. The extremely dry brush came right up to the edge of the west side of our tract, so the danger was very real. In fact, our street was blocked off by fire trucks, their hoses spread everywhere, and my nine year old Robby even climbed onto our roof, standing guard with our garden hose.

No one was allowed to enter the area, but Mary Jo's husband, Don, and his son Jim talked their way through, explaining that I was handicapped and had two young children with me. We all wore masks to keep from choking on the smoke, and our car was soon packed with our valuables, ready to leave should it prove necessary.

The fire raged all night, and our street pavement glowed red. Thankfully, it was contained later that next morning, but three hours after the containment, the hills on the east side of our house were on fire, and we were threatened once again. Again we went on alert, and again we did not have to evacuate, as the fire was finally extinguished. I was greatly relieved to have my home still intact and my children safe, but it was a horrible, frightening experience. Later it became known that someone had set fires all through the area. This is always a hazard of living in southern California.

Two years later, my divorce was final. I got my California teaching credentials and was hired by the Antelope Valley school district. My classroom was at Quartz Hill High School, and my students were special education students. I was the first special ed teacher the school had ever hired, so it was a new experience for them as well as for me.

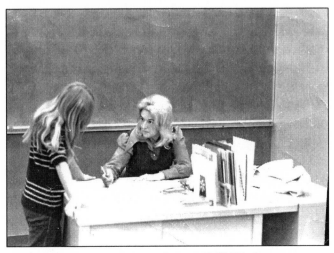

*In my class at Quartz Hill High*

Most of my students could barely read, and with the school year quickly approaching, there wasn't enough time to order and get the books needed for the class. I had to improvise, so I got some second-grade readers from a nearby elementary school to tide me over until I could get the other books. One student, however, insulted by the choice, pitched his book into the wastebasket and stormed out of class, angrily announcing, "I'm not reading this stuff." That was a most inauspicious beginning for a brand-new schoolteacher.

Many of my students were troubled kids from troubled backgrounds. Several boys from the inner city of Los Angeles had been in trouble with the law and now lived at Circle Y ranch. One afternoon after school, I went to my car to leave, only to find it gone. Two of these boys had taken my keys out of my purse and took off with my car to go visit an aunt in Los Angeles. They had tossed my wheelchair out of the car, thinking that would provide the clue to their identification. Needless to say, their plan didn't work, and they were caught and my vehicle returned.

Another of my students was a boy who was one of twelve children. He lived in a garage in Leona Valley, where it gets very cold in the winter. I visited his home and was saddened and shocked to see the small size of the house for such a large family and the garage where my student lived with no heat. On another occasion, I visited a boy's mother, who was totally drunk at ten o'clock in the morning. These children had experienced much hardship and depri-vation in their lives, like the girl from the hills of

Arkansas who had lived with her grandmother and was fourteen years old before she ever attended school. Such were the lives of my students.

My classroom had a kitchen where the students learned to prepare food. Each week I would take two students to the grocery store to help them learn how to choose fresh fruits and vegetable wisely. Beforehand, we made a menu, looked in the newspaper for sales, and planned a grocery list to fit our budget. At the store, we looked at unit prices and compared them for the best bargain. At Thanksgiving we prepared a complete meal with turkey and all the trimmings, and we asked our principal to share the meal with us.

This was an invaluable life experience for all the students, but more so for some than for others. Several boys had never shopped in a grocery store before, being familiar only with small shops and convenience stores. It showed them an entirely new and better way of doing things.

We also worked on the students' math skills. The students from my class baked cookies to sell to other students in the quad area of the school, handling all the selling and making of change. Learning how to balance a checkbook was also part of their instruction.

Teaching was hard work, but fulfilling. I was being productive while earning my own way and taking care of my children. It had taken me a while to get here, but all my hard work and effort had paid off. But another change was on the horizon.

# *Chapter 9*

*I* was getting ready for school, sitting on my bed, when a loud crack and a powerful rolling jolt shook my entire house. I truly thought my roof was going to crash down upon me. It was 6:01 a.m., February 9, 1971, and the 6.6 magnitude Sylmar earthquake, centered just three miles from my home, had struck. Renee was six years old, and she woke up to a corner cabinet falling on her. Robby yelled for me, and the three of us climbed over furniture to get out of the house. (The furniture was replaced, but the fear of earthquakes still haunts my daughter.) All the neighbors got together to put up tents; no one wanted to go back into their homes. It was four weeks before we stopped having 4.0 aftershocks and felt safe enough to return home. In the meantime, the kids and I stayed with my friend Bessie.

While staying at Bessie's house, I met an acquaintance of hers, Bill. Two days after I met him, he was at my door with a bag of oranges. He kept coming to see me, and we did lots of fun things. We went to the beach, took long drives into the mountains on week-ends, and camped on the Kern River for a week. We picnicked with the kids, and Bill even took Robby rock climbing on one of our outings. We spent all our time together, and we married ten months later.

I was so very happy. After all I had been through, I had a complete family again. I envisioned a family like the one I had grown up in. In those days, Sunday was always my favorite day of the week. Mom would put a roast in the oven to cook while we were at Mass. As we walked in the back door after church, we were greeted by the most delicious aroma. While Mom worked to get dinner ready, Daddy set up the card table in the living room. Mr. Gould, the man who worked for my dad, would come over, and after we had eaten, we would play canasta or pinochle all afternoon. So inviting was the atmosphere that I preferred staying home to going out with friends. I was hoping my marriage would be like that.

My new husband was an abalone diver and had a boat anchored in Morrow Bay. I was still teaching when we married, but at the end of the school year, the kids and I moved to Morrow Bay to be with Bill. We lived in a darling little house with lots of flowers and rosebushes, and the living room window over-looked the beautiful bay.

I enrolled both Robby and Renee in school for the next year and prepared for my wonderful new life in Morrow Bay. It was a beautiful town with lots of shops, and I placed my ceramic dolls and pottery on consignment in one of the shops. Robby got a paper route in town and began saving for a new bicycle. He often went to the pier near our house next to a little grocery store to put his trap into the water, hoping to catch a crab. I loved the quaintness of the town and the fresh sea air. Life seemed new, fresh, and good here.

All that changed one terrible night in October. I had been shopping, and as I entered the house and walked down the hallway, I heard voices coming from my son's room. Not thinking much about it, I opened the door to Robby's room to ask Bill for help in unbuttoning my dress. Stunned beyond description, I saw the man I had married molesting my eleven-year-old son. Frozen to the spot and hardly able to breathe, I calmly said, "Get out of the house, or I'll kill you."

I talked with my son to see if this had ever happened before. Robby assured me it hadn't, and I was relieved to know that. We talked a while longer, and when I was sure he was okay, I wandered into the dining room and then sat down by the window, gazing out at a beautiful pink rose.

I guess I was naïve, but I didn't really know these things happened—and certainly not in my own family. For the next two days, I spent most of my time sitting at the window, numb and overwhelmed. I didn't cry, and I didn't feel angry. I simply couldn't process what had happened. It was all too much, so I just sat and looked at that pink rose because it was the only beauty I could see.

From that moment on, I felt frantic in my own home. Wild thoughts tormented me: *Where's Bill? . . . Where are Robby and Renee? . . . What if Bill comes back and tries it again? . . . What do I do now?* On the third day, I knew I had to break this cycle of thought, so I called a therapist in San Louis Obispo and made an appointment. I did ask Bill to go with me, and he said he would; but when the time came, he backed out. I took my kids and went without him.

The doctor helped clarify my options. I had three choices, he said: keep things the same and stay with Bill, put my kids in a foster home and stay with Bill, or leave the marriage. The first two options were not really options to me, so I had no choice but to leave. I called my mother, informing her that I was leaving Bill and needed money. Without asking any questions, Mom sent me what I needed. I rented a U-Haul, and three days later my children and I were back in Canyon Country.

Fortunately, I still owned my home there. When I moved to Morrow Bay, I rented it out to a family, but they soon stopped paying their rent. Then a neighbor called to tell me the renters had left in the middle of the night. By the grace of God, I had an empty house to move back into. God was watching out for me, even in the bleakest of situations.

All the way home, I cried, heartbroken with the abrupt end of my fairy-tale life. I really did love Bill, but I knew I couldn't live with him. In those days, there wasn't the awareness of child molesters as there is now. Though I did leave Bill, I didn't call the police and have him arrested, which later became one of my biggest regrets.

Since it was October, the schools had already finished hiring, and no positions were available. In

January, I managed to find work at Palmdale High School as a long-term substitute. During one of my classes one day, I was showing a film that had a scene of the ocean. Memories of Morrow Bay came flooding into my mind, and before I knew it, I was crying in front of my class, much to my great mortification.

The next day as I was driving to Palmdale, I looked at myself in the rearview mirror and was shocked at my appearance. I had been crying almost every day for the last seven months now, and my face and eyes were so swollen that I didn't even look like myself. And on top of my physical appearance, my feelings and emotions were totally mixed up. I had wanted a family so badly, and I was still very much in love with my husband, but I knew I could not stay with him. He had done a hideous, despicable, and contemptible thing to my child; yet, I still loved him. I was sure something must be wrong with me to feel this way.

As I was driving to school that day, I realized I couldn't go on like this. I couldn't show up at school crying, but I didn't know what to do. Returning home, I called the school and told them that I couldn't come in because Renee had broken her arm (I have no idea where that came from). I then called my team teacher and told him I felt like I was in a box, with all my pieces broken and someone was trying to nail the box shut. Alarmed by my words, he called my neighbor and she started looking for me, fearing I was going to commit suicide.

I drove myself to Oliveview Hospital in San Fernando, but when I got there, I couldn't find the entry door. I found a phone booth and called the hospital. "Hello? I . . . I need help. Is there someone there to help me?" I haltingly asked.

"Ma'am," the kind voice on the other end began, "where are you? We'll come pick you up and get you the help you need."

"No, you don't need to do that," I protested. "I'm already here at the hospital . . . in the parking lot. I just can't find the door to get in. Just tell me where the door is, and I'll be fine."

"Stay right there. We'll be there in just one minute, and everything will be all right," the voice reassured.

True to their words, someone showed up and took me to a doctor. I don't remember much of our conversation, only that he asked me if I wanted to rest. That sounded so good to me. *Yes . . . rest . . . that's what I need,* my weary mind whispered.

The doctor asked if I wanted to go to a private hospital or to Camarillo. Not understanding the significance of the inquiry, I said I wanted a private hospital, only later discovering that Camarillo was a mental hospital. Thank God for watching over me while I made that choice!

My mother came to stay with my kids while I was in the hospital. During my two weeks there, the staff helped me understand that a person doesn't suddenly shut off love as if it were a water faucet. That was why I still had feelings for Bill. But the love was mixed with deep anger and a devastating sense of betrayal.

Gradually I began working through these conflicting emotions. One day I was lying on my hospital bed in my room and began fantasizing about a black stuffed chair in the corner. In my fantasy, the chair was Bill, and I stabbed it until the white stuffing came out. This was a turning point for me. Finally I felt like I could pull through this horrendous ordeal and move on.

After I left the hospital, I continued my counseling for months, and Rob also started counseling. By the time I was on an even keel, the new school year had started again, and I was hired as a substitute teacher for the Saugus school district. In addition, the county of Los Angeles hired me for substitute teaching. Substitute teaching worked wonderfully for me because I could be home soon after my kids arrived home from school. Slowly I began putting the pieces of my life back together.

# *Chapter 10*

$\mathcal{M}$onths later a new chapter in my life began when my friend Yvonne told me about Parents Without Partners, a group for single, divorced, and widowed parents. This organization was not only a group for adults in the same circumstance, but also one to provide activities for our kids. We had campouts, backyard barbeques, swimming parties, and other such fun-filled activities. For us single parents, it was a wonderful social group both for ourselves and for our children.

I became quite involved in the group and was the social director for a year. I had great fun arranging our many events. Planning the menu and ordering the food for dances was especially challenging. The New Year's Eve party was particularly challenging because it was open to the public, and I certainly didn't want to run out of food on a big occasion like that!

I loved dancing to the music of the bands we hired for these events. Slow dances were easy for me, but fast dances were harder and more tiring. If I held on to one hand of my partner, however, I was able to move my feet and body to the rhythm of the music. Best of all, when I was in the middle of the dancers, my leg brace wasn't even visible, and I looked like everyone else.

We often took trips to many different places, such as the Santa Anita racetrack and Hearst Castle, to name just two. We always had a great time, but I remember one trip in particular: river rafting on the south fork of the American River near Sacramento.

The thirty participants first rode a bus to the river and camped overnight before the expedition. We all slept together under one huge canopy. My friend Vi and other women helped me undress for bed, forming a circle around me and holding up blankets for privacy. The following morning, we clambered aboard five rafts and started down the river with our guides.

Everyone paddled, except for me. The guide instructed me to sit next to him and to hold on to him and the life jacket of the person sitting next to me. What a magnificent view of the mountains awaited us on both sides of the river as we floated slowly down the canyon! It was quiet, serene, and picture perfect. Suddenly the quiet was broken by loud yells coming from another raft. I looked up to see my friend Don in the river, dog-paddling, trying to keep his head above water to protect the cigarette in his mouth. He had been thrown in by the others in his raft. Just as he was pulled back into the raft, someone else was thrown into the water. In just a short time, everyone was being pulled in and others thrown out. I, of course, wasn't thrown in, but I got sopping wet, nonetheless. It was great fun.

Next on the agenda were water fights. The guides had brought buckets along, so we used them to scoop water out of the river and douse one another. We were so caught up in our hilarity that we didn't even notice when we hit the whitewater. Our guide yelled for everyone to row, instructing first one side then the other. My only job was to hold on tight, and that I did well! What an unforgettable adventure! I flipped up into the air and landed safely, only to be thrown from side to side in the raft.

But just as quickly as we had gone into the rapids, we emerged into calm water. We repeated this pattern several more times, and in the last set of rapids, I flipped up and came down hard on my bad leg. Because of my injury, I had to be carried piggy-back up to the bus at the end of the day. The guide wouldn't hear of me going the next day because he said these rapids were much rougher. But I was satis-fied: I had had my chance and shot the rapids!

The next event I planned for Parents Without Partners was a cruise. I thought this would be a great adventure, but I knew I couldn't afford it. When I talked to Faye, a travel agent who was also a friend of my sister's, she said that if I could get sixteen people to sign up for a Mexican cruise sailing on April 10, I could go for free. I was so excited, but as time passed, I had only twelve people who had actu-ally put their money down for the trip. I was very disappointed that I would not be going with them.

Then one day the phone rang, and I answered. I was greeted by my sister, Mary Jo. We made small talk for a couple of minutes, and then Mary Jo asked me, "What are you doing on April 10? Any special plans?"

I answered, "Oh, that's the day everyone else is going to Mexico. They're going to have a great time!"

"Well, so are you," she chuckled. "You're going too. I bought a ticket for you!" I was speechless and touched at her generosity and kindness.

The time for the cruise arrived, and we set sail on the *M. V. Stardancer.*

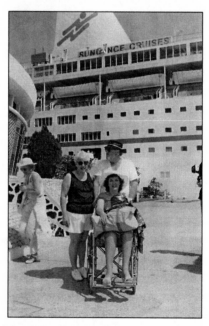

**Mary Jo, Don and myself on cruise**

We visited the Mexican cities of Mazatlán, Puerta Vallarta, and Cabo San Lucas. In Cabo San Lucas, I decided to stay on the ship while the others went into town. As I was sitting on the top deck, the captain of the ship came by and joined me. We talked for a while, and when I returned to my cabin, there was an envelope on the door. It was an invitation for me and my group to join him for cocktails in his cabin followed by lunch.

Arriving at his cabin, we immediately discovered that the door was too narrow for my wheelchair. Like a true gentleman, the Captain had one of his men take the door off its hinges so I could pass through.

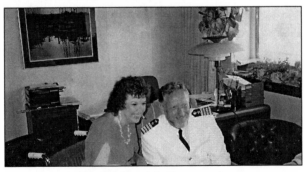

**Cocktails with the captain**

We chatted as he fixed drinks at his bar, and I browsed through one of his many books about ships. I mentioned my crossing on the ship I had taken to Europe twenty-five years earlier, and the captain looked through his books and found her story. Only five years after I had sailed on her, the *Johan Van Oldenbarnevelt* had sunk off the coast of Argentina in 1963. She had caught fire on a cruise from Southampton, England, and was abandoned with the loss of 128 lives. Later she capsized and sank.

We were very fortunate to be invited to the bridge. Not many people have a chance to do that. The view from the bridge of the ship was awesome, almost 180 degrees, and as I gazed at the water below, it was obvious how high up we were. Here at the ship's hub were screens that looked like large TVs set up in a semicircle with some men sitting and others standing in front of them. We talked to the senior officer a few minutes then went to lunch.

All in all, it was a wonderful trip. But too soon it was over, and we all returned to life as usual.

# *Chapter 11*

*I* continued participating in Parents Without Partners (PWP) and was greatly helped by the group discussions and professional speakers. Since the death of my second marriage, I had felt that I was failing as a parent, because my kids had no father in the home with them. With counseling, however, I came to realize that the three of us were a family, just as we were, and it was okay! That was a big revelation for me, something I really needed to know and believe.

I continued substitute teaching, and this time they sent me to an elementary school in Palmdale. But this particular school utilized bungalows for classrooms, and that meant steps. I knew I would not be able to maneuver the steps without help, so I asked some of the teachers if they would help me. Much to my surprise and dismay, they refused, saying they might hurt themselves. What made the whole thing even more disheartening was the fact that these were teachers of the handicapped.

When I talked to the county school office about the situation, they said that in the future they would send me only to places that didn't have steps. That would be very limiting, so I knew I had to find another way to earn a living if I couldn't resolve the issue with the steps. I did make a visit to the Fair Employment Practice Commission in downtown Los Angeles, which was created to eliminate discriminatory employment practices, but they said they couldn't help me.

I was forced to look for another way to support my family. The most important consideration was for me to be with my kids as much as possible. I wanted them to have my values and my outlook on life, and I knew that was possible only if I spent time with them.

While my employment issues were coming to a head, I was also having problems at home. Preteens and teenagers have been known to give their parents a rough time, and Rob was no exception. During his years in junior high school, I started having problems with him. The first inkling of trouble was when the school authorities showed up at my home one day to tell me that I had to get Rob to school. That was the first time I realized he had not been attending. After that, I drove him to school each day, but he simply waited until I left and then walked away. He absolutely refused to go to school.

Rob's school absences were causing quite a bit of trouble for both him and me. I talked to my counselor about it, and he advised me to send Rob to a boys' home. He recommended Pacific Lodge in Woodland

Hills, California. The home did not have any fences, and the boys were sent to the nearby public school, Parkman Junior High. The boys lived in dorms, and each dorm had an adult in charge. To motivate the boys toward acceptable behavior, there was a point system in place. If a boy gathered enough points, he was allowed to go to the movies or participate in excursions to the mall or beach, whatever was planned for that week. The boys who didn't earn enough points had to stay at the lodge while everyone else went.

The first week Rob was there, he decided to come home and started walking the twenty-mile trek from the city streets of Woodland Hills to San Fernando. To get home to Canyon Country, he had to cross a maze of freeways. Not knowing how to do that, Rob called me to pick him up. I did pick him up, but I drove him straight back to Pacific Lodge. That was an extremely difficult thing for me to do, but I had to do what was best for my son—even if he didn't understand it.

Rob was soon allowed to come home on weekends, and one weekend as we were traveling back to the lodge, he announced, "I'm not going in when we get there. I don't want to go back, and you can't make me."

Taken aback by his unexpected response, I began trying to reason with him, but to no avail. "You've got to go back, Rob. You know you do. You can't just sit in the car, and you can't go home with me. You've got to go in when we get there."

Not to be swayed, he insisted that he wouldn't go in, and I desperately pleaded with him to change his mind. "Please, Rob, can't you just do what you have to do? Just go in without causing any trouble. Can't you do that . . . please?" My pleading had no more effect on him than had my reasoning.

Arriving at the lodge, I found a counselor and told him Rob was refusing to come in. Quite nonchalantly, the counselor walked over to the car, leaned his head in the window, and said, "Come on, Dieguez. Let's go in."

Rob opened the door and went with him—just like that! No outburst, no grumbling, he just went! It took the air right out of me. I had been trying so hard, and then the counselor just said let's go and he went. Though happy with the outcome, I couldn't help but wonder how the counselor had done it.

A little later, Rob asked me what he had to do to come home. I told him he had to follow the rules of the lodge and earn grades no lower than a C. Determined to achieve his goal, he set to work and was later awarded a plaque recognizing him for attaining the most outstanding achievement of the year.

Praying my rosary and reading the words of a certain poem helped me through those times. The poem by Rudyard Kipling is entitled "If" and hung on the wall in my kitchen. I read it many, many times during those dark days, and the most inspirational lines for me were these:

> If you can force your heart and nerve and sinew
> To serve your turn long after they are gone,
> And so hold on when there is nothing in you
> Except the Will which says to them: "Hold on!"

Hold on I did, and God saw me through that time and many times thereafter when I needed strength beyond myself.

# *Chapter 12*

*A*s I was trying to figure out what type of job I should pursue next, my friend Yvonne invited me to her Tupperware party. The dealer hosting the party talked about selling Tupperware as a way to make money. I decided to give it a try, thinking that even if I earned only a little money, it would help. So I bought their blue suitcase full of wares and asked my neighbors Bessie and Jane to help me get my business off the ground. They graciously agreed to host parties, and Yvonne, too, offered her home. I organized the parties, demonstrated the Tupperware products, and then sold the items through catalogs and order forms. My Tupperware career was up and running!

Being a Tupperware dealer involves more than just demonstrating the product, as I soon discovered. After the demonstration at a party, I had to find women willing to host future parties. Each hostess agreed to invite her friends and family to a Tupperware party in her home, and in return, she would receive a hostess gift, which could be anything from a Crock-Pot to an electric skillet. One party usually led to another, and before long I was having lots of parties.

After I had recruited three dealers and filled a date book with three to five parties a week, I was promoted from dealer to manager. As manager, I received an additional commission on my unit, and I was responsible for training my dealers, motivating them, and getting them to sales rallies. Even better than the commission, however, was the Pontiac company car I now drove. Not having a car payment or insurance payment was great, and I got a new car every several years.

My business really thrived. At one point, I had sixteen dealers in my unit. When my dealers recruited three dealers of their own, they were then promoted to manager. In this way, the network grew and flourished. During my time in Tupperware, I was able to promote five managers of my own.

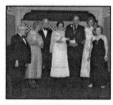

**Promoting a Tupperware manager**

It was physically demanding work, however, and I was exhausted at the end of each day. At twelve years old, Renee was a big help, carrying the suitcases into and out of the houses and setting up the tables for me. I did my demonstrations, and more people signed up to host more parties. Surprisingly, it wasn't hard to keep finding new hosts and new groups of people to show the products to.

Tupperware conventions, also called Jubilees, were held once a year, and as a manager, I attended all of them. Sometimes they were held in Utah, but regardless of the location, there was usually a theme for which we all dressed accordingly. My distributorship, VerVon Sales, always played a big role in these conventions, so it was a great fun time for us. Many, many prizes were awarded, and one of my most special prizes was the white canopied bedroom set I won for my daughter. She deserved it, with all the help she had given me.

The years rolled by, and eventually I was having so many parties and my garage was so full of product that I had to hire my neighbor to do all the packing. Even my son got into the act and became a Tupperware dealer for a short time. All the women loved Rob, so he had no problem booking new parties. His friendliness and good looks made him a big hit.

After being in Tupperware for six years, I was feeling very tired and stressed. My busy pace of life seemed to be catching up with me. My doctor, thinking I might be having heart problems, ordered me to wear a Holter monitor, a portable device for continuous monitoring of the electrical activity of the heart.

Also, as a result of a sleep study he ordered for me, he prescribed a BiPap. This is a machine that forces air through a mask and into a person's lungs and can be set at one pressure for inhaling and another for exhaling. With these dual settings, the BiPap allowed me to get more air in and out of my lungs without the natural muscular effort that's normally required. It works on the same premise as the iron lung, but it is much more comfortable. So well did it work that I've been wearing it every night for twenty-seven years now.

Much to my relief, the Holter monitor revealed no problem with my heart, but shortly after, I had a new problem: I had breast cancer. When the doctor showed me the X-ray, I didn't feel particularly nervous or upset. I just calmly and stoically took it all in. Later, however, I was having lunch with Yvonne and telling her about it. As I lifted my coffee cup to my mouth, you could hear the click-clicking of the cup against my teeth. I guess I was more shaken then I realized.

I decided to go to the UCLA oncology department for a second opinion. They performed a biopsy, and the results were the same—cancer. Thankfully, it was in the early stages, but as a precaution, I had a complete mastectomy and all my lymph nodes removed as well. The doctors believed my cancer was fueled by high amounts of estrogen, so to further strengthen my recovery, they recommended I have a complete, or radical, hysterectomy.

After a year, I felt I had adjusted to my mastectomy to the point where I could pursue breast reconstructive surgery. The UCLA doctors did a procedure called the Latissimus Dorsi flap. This procedure pulls muscle, fat, and skin from the upper back to the chest to create a breast mound; the muscle then covers a silicone prosthesis used in the process.

A year later, my sister and I were vacationing in a hotel in Lake Arrowhead. I was telling her that it felt like my body was turning to stone. Turning my arms one way then the other was slow and very difficult. Mary Jo listened intently and then remarked that she had read of some women having trouble with silicone prostheses. The article explained that oils gradually leach out of the shells and over time enter body tissues. I wondered if that could be my problem and decided to have the implant removed. I followed up with my decision, and afterward I no longer had that frozen feeling.

But all the surgeries had sapped my strength, and I knew I wouldn't be able to do Tupperware parties anymore. It was time to see what the next phase of my life would bring.

# *Chapter 13*

*G*iving up my Tupperware career, I managed to find a part-time job in the library at the College of the Canyons in Valencia. Since I was still recovering from my surgeries, the librarian allowed me to work only when I felt well. Six months later, however, the library lost its "soft money," a term used for monies that must be applied for each year. When it's gone, there isn't any more until the next year. What that meant for me was that I was out of work again, but I heard about a job opening in the college's career center and applied. I had never heard of a career center, but the ten-hour workweek was just what I needed. I was still trying to rebuild my stamina, and that time frame was as much as I could handle.

The so-called career center consisted of a small room with two computers, two desks, and lots of boxes jammed in the back. My immediate boss worked a twenty-hour week. Because we were financed by soft money, she feared our money would soon be cut, so several months later she opted to leave. The dean then put me in charge.

Joan Jacobson was a career counselor at the college, and she kindly took me under her wing. A wonderful mentor, she guided me through the next eight years, helping me put together a career package for students. As part of my responsibilities, I went to classes to present a very short talk about what the center had to offer. After identifying two careers of interest, students would explore those options and then follow up with one of the counselors.

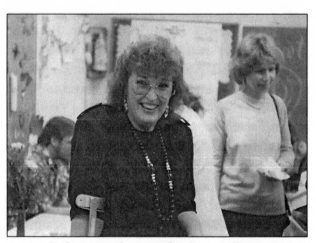

**Helping students at the Career Center**

Within a year I was full-time, and now we had five computers with career assessment software to help identify careers of interest and other software to provide information regarding specific careers. The center gradually expanded until we took up one-third of the building's first floor with our computers, career library, and job-placement section. Soon I had seven part-time people working for me. Once a year we hosted a job fair, which the nearby businesses attended.

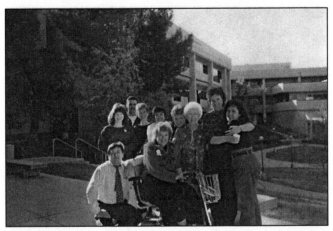

*Career Center staff & the dean of Student Services*

When there were job cutbacks in the industrial center I approached the president of the college with the idea of offering the same career package for non-students for a nominal fee. She thought it was a good idea and gave me permission to proceed but instructed me to offer it through the on campus community extension program.

While I was busy adapting to all the changes in my career, my life at home was changing too. Rob joined the U.S. Army Reserves and went to Alabama for his basic training. Although he was given the option of going into the regular army, he decided to stay in the reserves, which he did for six years. After returning home, Rob enrolled at the sheriff's academy in Los Angeles and lived with me until he had saved enough money to buy a mobile home nearby.

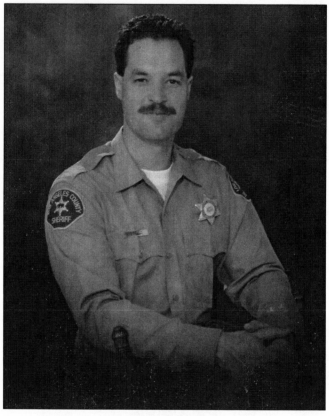

*Deputy Dieguez*

He was starting a new period in his life, and I was very proud of him. Nevertheless, I will admit that it was hard on me when he left home. Although Renée was still there, it was lonely without Rob, and

I realized it wouldn't be long before Renee would be leaving home too.

Two years later, Rob bought a home in Palmdale. He married and soon had two beautiful children, Sarah and Robbie. Today his daughter is a Los Angeles deputy sheriff, and his son is in the Air Force Special Forces. Unfortunately, his marriage lasted only a few years.

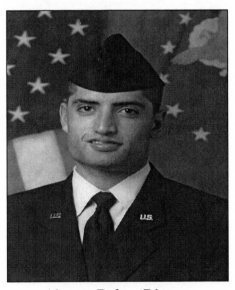

***Airman Robert Dieguez***

A number of years later, he met and married Oanh, a stunning beauty, a lady, and a good friend. After twenty-two years as a Los Angeles deputy sheriff, Rob finally retired. But he had made a difference in his career, as evidenced by the following story: During his time as a deputy, Rob was sent on a call where a six-year-old girl had been molested. Recalling his own childhood, Rob empathized with the child, confiding in her that the same thing had happened to him when he was young. The following is an excerpt from a letter the girl's mother sent to Rob's commanding officer after the incident:

That morning a mother's worst nightmare happened. I found out that my little innocent, beautiful daughter had been molested. You took a delicate situation and made the best out of it. You were so wonderful in making my daughter feel at ease before and during the interview. I have written to your commanding officer to express my appreciation for your compassion and kindness. I wish there were more people like you in the world and on the police force.

As time went on, it became too difficult for me to walk up the three-inch step into my home. I heard of a group from Los Angeles County that helped the handicapped and elderly with problems in their homes, and I applied to them for help. To my delight, three men came to my house and poured a concrete ramp for me, thus bypassing the need for me to maneuver the step. What a blessing those men were, and what a relief it was not to have to worry anymore about getting into my house!

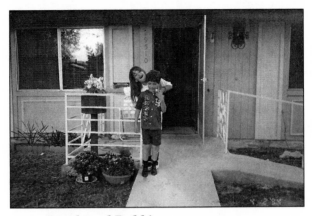

**Sarah and Robbie on my new ramp**

Changes were going on with Renee too, some good and some not so good. As she approached eighteen, Renee bought her first car, a Gremlin. She had saved her money and paid all of 350 dollars for it, but it was hers.

Renee worked at Magic Mountain, an amusement park near our home. She ran the basket shop by herself, and I was very proud of her. One Sunday in September, she left for work as usual. About noon that day, a manager from the park called to ask if Renee was okay, because she had not shown up for work. Worried sick, I feared something terrible had happened to her. Finally, around five o'clock, Renee sauntered into the house, oblivious to what I had been through that day.

I, of course, was relieved to see her and so thankful that she was safe, but I knew I had a problem on my hands. Calmly I greeted my daughter, "Hi, Renee.

Where have you been all day?" I kept my voice casual and pleasant.

"Oh, you know, just the usual. I've been working all day," she answered.

"Were you busy today, what with all the rain we had?" I queried further, letting her walk further into the trap.

"No, it was slow. Like you said, it rained all day; that always keeps people at home."

I had had enough and revealed the truth. "Well, maybe you should stay home a little more yourself. Then when your manager calls to ask why you're not at work, you can explain for yourself."

Renee just stood there, not saying anything until I wrapped up my speech with, "Since you weren't honest, you can't have the car for two weeks."

"That's not fair, Mom. It's just not fair. Besides, it's my car, and you can't take it away from me."

"Well, you're wrong there, young lady. I *have* taken it away from you—for two weeks."

"Then I'm out of here. I am not going to stay someplace where I'm treated like a child. I'm moving out!"

"Fine . . . okay . . . go for it then," I countered, not believing for a minute she would go through with it. At the most, I thought perhaps she would go to her girlfriend's house and come home the next day.

Well, Renee did leave, but she did not go to her girlfriend's. Instead, she moved in with a boyfriend I didn't even know she had! I was shocked and devastated, so afraid she was heading in the wrong direction, but I knew I had to count on her inner set of values and good sense. Since she was just a few months short of turning eighteen, it was pointless to pick her up and force her to return home as though she were a wayward thirteen-year-old. I could do nothing but hope and pray for the best.

Renee stayed with her boyfriend for a year but then decided on her own that this was not what she wanted. She moved out and rented a room for two hundred dollars from a friend. With this change in her living arrangements, I saw an opportunity for her to come home. I made her an offer she couldn't refuse. "If you move back home and pay me only fifty dollars a month as rent, you would have enough money to buy a brand-new car." Two weeks later, my daughter moved home. Together we went to the car dealer, and Renee bought a new Toyota. Our relationship, too, was new, and slowly we rebuilt it.

While Renee was in high school, she volunteered at the local hospital as a candy striper.

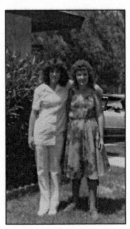

**Renee in candy stripe uniform**

She thought she wanted to be a registered nurse, and actually working in a hospital helped her make a positive decision. College of the Canyons did offer a nursing program, but I didn't have the funds to finance her education. After her graduation from high school, I suggested she apply for scholarships from benevolent clubs in our area, such as our local Rotary or Elks clubs. My dad, her grandfather, had been a member of the Elks in Warrensburg before he passed away, and I thought that might help.

Renee wrote a letter to the Elks and referred to her grandfather. Fortunately, I proofread the letter before she sent it and laughingly suggested she refer to her grandfather as a "deceased Elk"—not a "diseased" one! She took my advice and then mailed the letter. Only two weeks later, a member of the Elks stood at our door informing us that they were awarding Renee a full scholarship to the nursing program.

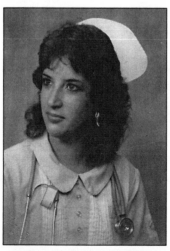

**Renee Dieguez RN**

A few years later, Renee traded her car for a Nissan Pathfinder. Time was flying by, and I knew it wouldn't be long before she would be on her own. In the meantime, I wanted to spend as much fun time with her as possible, so the two of us started traveling together in her Pathfinder. Every weekend we went somewhere, and we fit in as many vacations as our schedules would allow.

We had everything we needed in that Pathfinder, even though it was a bare-bones vehicle with no backseat. I got the idea to cut a piece of foam to fit in the flat area in the back where we could place our sleeping bags and have our own "bedroom." I even sewed little curtains to fit over the windows so we could have privacy at night. When evening came, we would tape them up, and then before setting out the next day, we would take them down.

The Grand Canyon was one of the first trips Renee and I took together. We packed a suitcase, put the ice chest in the Pathfinder, and washed Stashly, Renee's big Labrador retriever. The first night we stayed at Black Bart's RV Park, Steakhouse, and Saloon in Flagstaff, Arizona. The waiters and waitresses from the Arizona University music department not only served food but also entertained with a musical revue of old-time favorites, a delightful surprise to us.

We left the restaurant, and Renee pushed my chair back to the RV Park. In order for me to get into the back of the Pathfinder to sleep, Renee and I had devised an ingenious plan. First, Renee would crawl into the back while I remain seated in the front. Next, she would hook her arms under my arms and pull while I pushed on the dash with my good foot. Finally, the momentum would propel me over the seat, and both Renee and I would land in a heap in the back. I'm sure we must have looked comical, but it worked for us! When morning came, I could simply slide out the back end of the Pathfinder and into my wheelchair.

The next morning we left for the Grand Canyon. This natural wonder is so immense and so inspirational that there is no way to put into plain words the power of the landscape. The only way to realize it is to see it in person. As a child of ten, I had visited the canyon and, like so many others, ridden a donkey down into it. The experience had always stayed with me, and when I had children of my own, I always hoped to share this magnificent display of nature with them. By the time Renee and I took our trip, Rob had already moved from home, but at least I was able to share it with my daughter.

Another memorable trip was to Taos, New Mexico. Taos Pueblo, a living Native American community and a national historic landmark, is known for being one of the most secretive and conservative pueblos in the country. The multistoried adobe buildings have been inhabited for over one thousand years. Driving into the village, I felt like I was in a time warp. We paid a fee to enter and were given strict instructions about what to do and what not to do. We were limited as to where we could go and had to stay in our car. There could be no stopping, and no photography was allowed. Just as we were leaving, Renee suddenly jumped out of the car, exclaiming, "Mom, quick, take my picture!"

"Renee, are you crazy? Get back in here," I yelled. But I soon switched tactics and took the picture, realizing it was faster to snap the picture and hope the camera wasn't confiscated than to argue with her.

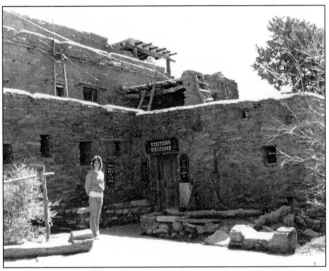

***Renee at Taos***

Driving on, I was facinated by a reddish brown adobe building. Several men were patching it as we drove by, using a material made from sand, clay, and water, with some kind of sticks or straw mixed in. This material was then shaped by hand into bricks. Several men did this every single day of every year, as some part of the structure was in constant need of repair.

The river running through the pueblo serves as the primary source for drinking and cooking water for the residents of the village. Electricity, running water, and indoor plumbing are strictly prohibited. At the time of our visit, 150 people still lived there.

From New Mexico, we traveled to Durango, Colorado, and found a beautiful campground next to the Animas River. We decided to stay at the campground several days and take a side trip to Silverton via the Durango & Silverton Narrow Gauge Railroad. This train winds through spectacular, breathtaking canyons and crosses on high trestles. The train hugs the mountain, and as we came around a curve, I saw the framework of a trestle ahead. With its slanted supports and horizontal crosspieces, it rose quite high from the canyon floor.

The history of the excursion was mind-boggling; we were traveling on a coal-fired, steam-powered locomotive on the same tracks miners, cowboys, and settlers of the Old West had traveled on one hundred years before. Although the line was constructed for the strictly utilitarian purpose of hauling silver and gold ore from the mountains, its view was truly spectacular.

There were a number of homes in these mountains that could be accessed only by foot or train. As the train approached certain designated places, it would slow down so that people from the back country could flag the train down to board or to send mail. The conductor gave Renée his conductor's hat and asked her to stick her head out the window and look ahead to see if anyone was waving for the train to stop.

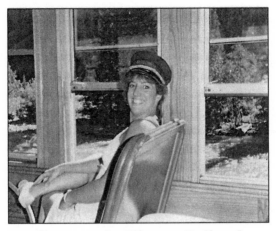

***Renee on the Silverton Railroad***

If no one was there, we zipped on by. Finally, we arrived in Silverton, the town of boom or bust, a town of hundreds of miners all wanting to be the "silver king" of Colorado. A ghost town for years, Silverton was later revived for tourism.

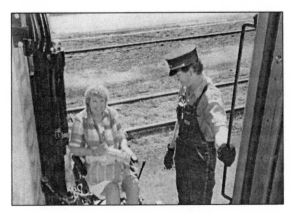

***All aboard***

Traveling on through Colorado, Renee and I arrived in Grand Lake, the last town before Trail Ridge Road. I recalled traveling this same road with my mother once, so Renee and I decided to travel the same route. I guess I didn't remember how scary that road is. What a mistake that turned out to be!

Only two lanes wide, Trail Ridge Road is the highest continuous highway in the United States. At ten thousand feet, it became more difficult for us to breathe. The landscape reminded me of the Arctic tundra, barren and treeless. At the top the road rose above eleven thousand feet, and at one point, our elevation topped twelve thousand feet. The wind was whipping furiously and rocking our van as we traversed the road. Renee was gripping the wheel tightly, and we were both scared to death. She started crying, but I had no time to comfort her. All I could say was, "Stop crying, or you won't see the road." That common-sense instruction did seem to calm her, but she remarked, "This is as close to heaven as I want to get!" Inwardly, I agreed.

On another trip one summer, we went to Montana and Wyoming and stayed at a campsite on the west side of Yellowstone National Park. We drove inside to the most famous geyser in the park, and perhaps the world: Old Faithful. At approximately seventy-four-minute intervals every day, the geyser erupts. First you hear a gurgling noise, then the spray starts spitting, and suddenly the spray shoots up ten to twelve stories high. It was a remarkable sight.

We decided to go to the Lake Yellowstone Hotel for lunch that day. When we were almost finished eating, we heard talk of a black bear roaming down the main street of a nearby village. Renee was so excited that nothing would do but to immediately leave to go see it. Hurriedly she got me into the car, threw my wheelchair in the back, and off we went. We arrived just in time to see the rangers putting the bear into a contained trailer. They had already tranquilized and marked it and were taking it to the high country for release. At least Renee got to see the bear's rear end as the rangers were loading it! We got a good laugh out of that.

Forest fires occur in the park each year; in the large forest fires of 1988, nearly one-third of the park was burned. Our campsite was located at the west entrance to Yellowstone Park, so we had to pass through that area. By now it was evening, and with no moon it was pitch-black and very spooky as the car's headlights illuminated the dead remains of the burned forest on each side of the road. Renee was driving, and I was tense, leaning forward to stare out the front window. "Renee," I said, "we haven't seen a car for miles. I don't like being out here all alone. Are you sure we're going the right way?"

Renee didn't answer but just kept driving. Unknown to me, she was busy sliding her hand along the back of the seat toward me. I didn't notice a thing until she suddenly tapped me on my back. To her great delight, I let loose with a scream that I'm sure could be heard clear across the park! Thanks to my mischievous daughter, I was sure some swirly monster had attacked me.

Renee and I continued our travels together, treasuring this special time we shared. Some weekends and holidays we would just get into her van and go. We loved it, so much so that before long I bought a little trailer that we could hook up to her Pathfinder. Now we were really going places!

It was a small trailer, but just the right size for the two of us. It had no air conditioner, but it did have a heater, and best of all, it had a large bathroom with a bathtub. Since I am unable to rise from a regular-height toilet seat, we adapted the toilet to a greater height by taking it out and building a box structure under it. (In order to get out of any seat by myself, it must be built up or rise mechanically.)

On one of our trips, we traveled up the West Coast through Oregon and on to Washington State. We ferried over to Vancouver Island and toured the beautiful Butchart Gardens, fifty acres of the most spectacular floral displays imaginable. Fifty gardeners constantly plant, prune and tend these magnificent gardens.

Growing season was at its peak when we visited. What a delicious treat for the senses it was! The vibrant color of thousands of red tulips popping up through a carpet of white alyssum was incredibly impressive. We followed a meandering path over little bridges winding through manicured lawns, enveloped by the wonderful fragrance of the rainbow mix of sweet peas. Fountains surrounded by yellow black-eyed Susans and tall snapdragons dotted the landscape. A wild brilliance and kaleidoscope of color awaited us at every turn.

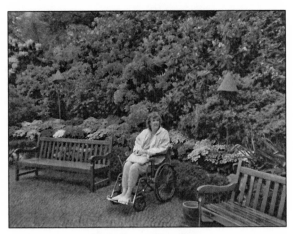

**Butchart Gardens**

After the day spent at the gardens, we ferried back to British Columbia, drove down to Washington, and parked our trailer beside a stream in a KOA campground. Parking our trailer next to the stream, we took off for the interior of Canada. We were traveling on a new, wide highway to Kamloops, British Columbia, but there was no gas station or stop for seventy-five miles.

As the trip wore on, Renee grew very tired. Also, it was getting dark, so we decided to stop in Merrit, the first town coming up. Arriving in the city, we couldn't find any place to stay, however, because it was a Canadian holiday, Victoria Day. All the hotels and motels were completely booked.

Finally, at the edge of the town, we saw a vacancy sign. Anxious to obtain the room and celebrating our good fortune at finding it, Renee hurried into the motel office. But after looking at the room, she hopped back into the car and said, "Nope, I think this is a place that rents by the hour! We either sleep in the car or keep moving."

So we kept moving, finally arriving in Kamloops an hour and a half later. Exhausted beyond description, we found a room in the Kamloops Hotel, which had converted a meeting room into a hotel room by putting a couple of beds in it. But that didn't matter to us; we were overjoyed just to have a decent place to lay our heads.

Heading back to the States, we stopped at Hell's Gate on the Fraser River. Renee wanted to go deep into the gorge on an air tram. A large electric motor located at the bottom of the tramway pulls one cabin down while using that cabin's weight to help pull the other cabin up. We would not only be going down into the gorge, but we would also be going across the river.

After my experience in Austria years earlier, I was scared to death to even think about boarding the tram. I had two choices: go down with Renee, or stay by myself at the top. Making my decision, I thought, *If we crash, at least we'll die together.* With that, we boarded the tram, and although I was scared, the ride was not nearly as bad as the one in Austria. When we got down into the gorge, I even took a few steps on the suspension bridge to gaze at the fury of the river below.

On our outings, we usually stayed at KOA campgrounds because I felt they were clean and safe. In western Washington, Renee was unhooking our trailer while I was talking to an older man in the next campsite. He said I should plug in my electrical cord on the opposite side of the trailer, and I said I would tell my daughter. Astonished, he asked, "You mean, you don't have a man with you?" He couldn't believe a young girl and a handicapped woman were traveling alone. I don't think I realized just how different we were, especially for that time. As far as Renee and I were concerned, we were just a mother and daughter enjoying life the best way we knew how.

As we were traveling along the Columbia River, we saw a paddle wheeler getting ready for a short cruise. It was about to depart, but we were able to purchase tickets at the last minute. I found it fascinating to travel the same river that Lewis and Clark had seen when they cut through the Cascade Mountains between Oregon and Washington.

Local natives were fishing the river the way they had done for centuries. We saw an eagle diving into the water, grabbing a fish and flying straight up into the air with the fish hanging from its mouth. Seconds before the plank was raised, a nice-looking young man near Renee's age boarded, and the two of them talked to each other during the entire cruise. The three of us made plans to meet again at the salmon locks at the Bonneville Dam, our next stop.

Franklin D. Roosevelt had signed the bill for the construction of the dam as a public works projects during the Depression. The dam enables the salmon to pass around barriers by swimming and leaping up a series of relatively low steps or ladders into the waters on the other side. The water falling over the steps has to be strong enough to attract the fish to the ladder, but it can't be so strong that it washes them back downstream or exhausts them to the point that they can't continue upriver.

Through a viewing glass constructed especially for visitors, Renee, the young man, and I watched the salmon hurtling up the fish ladder. Off the main room, a woman sat at a desk, counting each fish as it passed by her section of the ladder. We also watched a movie about the building of the dam. Hundreds of men from all parts of the country had participated in its construction. America was in the Great Depression, and the dam's construction provided jobs, even if far from home.

One part of the movie featured a waitress who was asked to be married by one of the construction men after only one date. I looked at Renee sitting next to the young man, whose name was Stacey, and thought, *Wouldn't it be funny if that happened to Renee?* I could tell they enjoyed each other's company, so after our visit to the locks, I took Renee aside and said, "Renee, ask Stacey over to our campground for dinner."

"Mother, I couldn't do that!" Renee exclaimed.

"Okay, I will then," I answered, and I did! Stacey was traveling alone on his way back to the Silicone Valley after having visited his grandmother, and he eagerly accepted my dinner invitation. By the time dinner was over, it was growing dark, and Stacey got his tent out from his car and pitched it next to our trailer. The next day, he caravanned down the coast with us. Later I remember thinking, *Oh my, I think we just picked up a man!* But all's well that ends well, as the old saying goes. Two months later, Stacey and my daughter were engaged, and eight months later they were married. That was seventeen years and two children ago.

# Chapter 14

*I*n the summer of 1992, Renee, Mary Jo, and I went on a southern Caribbean cruise.

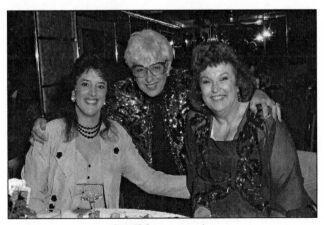

***Caribbean cruise***

One of our shore excursions was on the island of Martinique. I asked the person in charge of the excursions if I could have help going down the steps. He assured me that it was no problem and called for a worker to come and help me. I was sitting in my wheelchair, and the man stooped down, braced his back to the back of my chair, and lifted me like a bale of hay!

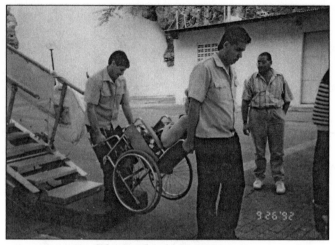

*Please don't say – oops*

As we approached the doorway, I warily looked down at all those steep steps we were going to have to take. The man was undeterred and started down, but I was terrified, thrust into the air with the ship's handrail out of reach and the water far, far below. I simply closed my eyes and prayed; what else could I do? I will admit, I had a couple of drinks before he carried me back up at the end of the excursion.

After docking in Barbados, we hired a cab to take us around the island. We didn't want to go on the regular sightseeing tour with everyone else. Our driver took us to a little out-of-the-way outdoor pub at the other end of the island. We each had a rum punch drink with lunch—just one rum punch, and all three of us were pretty giddy. We even had a lady on the beach come into the pub to put colored beads and corn rows in our hair.

For another cruise, an Alaskan cruise, I flew from Portland, Oregon, to Vancouver, British Columbia, to meet my sister, her husband, and Jim, their son. I was rooming with my nephew in a handicapped cabin so he could help me. That night when we were getting ready for bed, Jim had the cabin boy make up the couch. The cabin boy was upset because he thought we were a couple having an argument the first night of our cruise!

Jim was such a help to me. He helped me to get in and out of bed and in and out of the shower. To shower, I would put on a shift, and then Jim would scoot me from my chair to the shower chair. I then took off my shift for showering and put it back on when finished. In that way, I retained my privacy but got the necessary help.

The cruise was magnificent. Such awesome, majestic beauty surrounded us in the landscapes of glaciers and towering mountains. Sitting in the observation room, we all ran to the windows to see whales when some were spotted. Several of them flipped entirely out of the water, twisted in the air, and landed with a smack on their sides. What a sight!

In Juneau we traveled the fifty miles to Glacier Bay National Park and Preserve. Jim and I were on the deck looking at a glacier when I said it would be years before it would calve icebergs into the bay. Not even two minutes later, a huge chunk of ice dropped into the water. Well, so much for my analysis!

Another trip involved some of my family and friends who got together and rented a condo on Hawaii's Big Island. My sister, her husband, and Rosemarie, my friend from work, decided we should get first-class tickets for the flight. Normally when I travel, if an airport doesn't have a Jetway, I must board the airplane by being transferred from my scooter to a piece of equipment that looks like a dolly with a seat on it. I sit, cross my arms, and get both my arms and legs strapped down. While one person stays at my back, two others lift the front as they bump me up the steps into the airplane, squeeze me down the aisle, and lift me into my seat. My scooter is then stored in the luggage hold.

With the first-class ticket to Hawaii, however, I was traveling on a wide-bodied plane and able to drive my scooter into the plane and slide off into my seat. I was seated in the front row, and before me was a large banquet table laden with fruits and orchids. What service! The flight attendants were bustling about, pouring drinks and serving us a full course meal on china plates. Always before, I had been accustomed to half a sandwich on a paper plate! The trip over was wonderful, and when we disembarked in Hawaii, we were each greeted with the requisite leis for our necks.

The condo we rented was equipped for the disabled. It had a bathtub so large that at least ten people could have gotten into it! But I wasn't able to use it, so the ladies took me to the walk-in showers near the pool. One would stand guard while the others helped me disrobe. Wearing their bathing suits, they actually took a shower with me.

One of our excursions was with a tour group for snorkeling. The guide helped me put on the diving mask and ease into the brilliant, clear water. My sister was astonished to see my legs move. Water, however, gave me buoyancy, and free of the effects of gravity, I could move more easily.

Snorkeling was a wonderful opportunity to see underwater life in a natural setting. It was a different world, full of all sizes and colors of fish with constant movement. When the men from the boat carried me out of the water and up the steps, I looked at my chest and was flabbergasted. After being in the water, my left breast prosthesis (made of bagged rice) had swollen to twice the size of the other. It was quite a sight, as you might imagine!

On Sunday my sister and I went to Mass and discovered they were having a special multiethnic service in honor of Father Damien of Belgium, who had taken care of the lepers of Molokai. This great man spent sixteen years in the living graveyard that was Molokai, where he died of leprosy at the age of forty-nine.

On the island of Molokai, Father Damien lived among eight thousand people who had been banished there during the epidemic of the 1850s. He was originally buried on Molokai, but in 1936 the Belgian government asked for the return of his body, which was granted. The people of Molokai, however, had always wanted at least some part of Father Damien to be buried on the island. At this special multiethnic Mass, a relic bone from his right hand was being reinterred in the empty grave beside the small chapel of St. Philomena in Kalaupapa.

The procession began with islanders dressed in native garb and blowing a conch shell, which emitted a loud, distinctive sound as ceremonial fanfare. Women wearing muumuus and kuku'i nut necklaces comprised the honor guard for the relic. Portuguese in their native costumes played their guitars, and Hawaiian girls danced the hula to the words of the homily. In 1995 Pope John Paul II beatified Father Damien, leaving but one step remaining toward sainthood. That mark will be reached at a ceremony in the Vatican on October of 2009, when Pope Benedict XVI presides over the canonization of Father Damien de Veuster.

# *Chapter 15*

*I* had a friend that I wanted to give a special gift to one Christmas. After giving it much thought, I decided to paint a picture, but something more than a flower or a landscape. I wanted to paint a nude. My next-door neighbor took painting lessons, so I talked to her about it. She tried to dissuade me from it, pointing out that you don't start painting by taking on something as challenging as a nude. But I knew that's what I wanted.

My neighbor directed me to her painting instructor, Beverly, who had published a book of paintings. I thought she was the perfect person to help me. I bought a three-by-two-foot canvas and completed a rough sketch. I painted a woman holding a royal blue cloth up to her breasts. She was completely covered, except for her sides.

In the end result, the cloth was very beautiful, the body okay, and Beverly did the hands for me. It was a good try, but I realized I had better stick to flowers and landscapes.

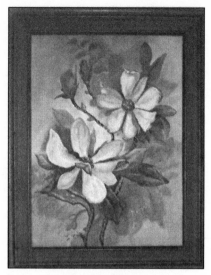

**Magnolia blossoms**

I enjoyed my new hobby and continued painting for several years, selling or giving away all but three of my creations. One of the portraits I did was of a friend of mine's two-year-old son.

Another of my ventures involved horseback riding, which I was able to do through Heads Up, a nonprofit organization dedicated to providing therapeutic riding for disabled children and adults. I had ridden horses before I got polio, so I was very excited to get on a horse again. In order to mount, I was lifted up to sit on a stack of hay. From there, I was able to get my leg over the horse's back and sit on him. He was so much bigger than I remembered horses being! At least two volunteers were with me at all times, and they walked me around the track several times, one on each side.

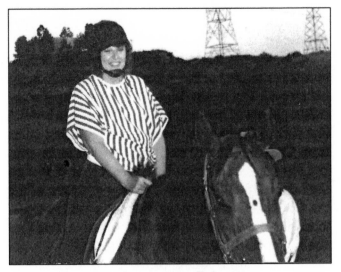

***Another accomplishment***

While I was busy learning new things, I began noticing some disturbing things in my body. At this point, I had been employed at the college in the career center for seven years. The changes were gradual, but insidious. For instance, I had always been able to step onto a curb by putting my good leg on it and then leaning over the car hood as I swung my bad leg up. I couldn't do that anymore. I had always been able to walk from the parking lot to my office, but that, too, was getting difficult. Before I left home for work, I would call the disabled center at school for someone to meet me, but sometimes they forgot about my request. At those times, I just had to stay patient until someone would notice my absence and ask, "Where's Marge?" Then the dean's secretary would rush out with the wheelchair to get me. Sooner or later, someone always showed up.

With my physical limitations increasing, it soon became necessary to buy a power scooter to help me get around. But it was becoming increasingly difficult to get out of my van. When my daughter had her first child, I drove by myself the three hundred miles from Canyon Country to San Francisco to be with her. By the time I arrived at the hospital, I was so tired and stiff that I couldn't get my chair out of the car. I had to ask a person walking by, a total stranger, to help me. I decided it was time to buy a modified van so I could be totally independent.

Because of my weak hands, it was necessary to buy a van with extremely sensitive steering, but the brakes and gas pedal could be normal. A ramp was sandwiched between the undercarriage and floorboard and emerged from the side door. It dropped to the ground and allowed me to back myself into the van. The driver's seat could be turned sideways so I could slide into it. A lever made it possible for me to turn the seat back into the driving position. Now I was independent, and it was glorious!

In my eighth year at the college, my legs were growing noticeably weaker. One day when I tried to get out of the shower, my legs wouldn't move at all, much to my dismay. Thankfully, my neighbor was there and called the paramedics. They had to carry me out to my bed. After I rested, I was able to get into my chair again, but I was disturbed by the episode.

Not long after that, I tried to stand but fell. My next-door neighbor rushed over and put me back into my chair. In an effort to prevent more falls, I started sliding from my bed to my chair. I bought a slick material and hemmed fifteen-by-twelve-inch pieces to help me slide more easily. I had come up with this idea during an airplane flight. Because of the rough cloth of my seat, I had been unable to move the entire trip—not even a slight wiggle. It was very painful, so when I got home, I made "sliders" to help me shift my position, even if only slightly. Now I put these sliders to use at home.

It soon became obvious to me that a forty-hour workweek was just too much. When I got home in the evenings, I lacked the energy and strength to cook for myself. All my physical reserves were poured into work, and I had nothing left over at the end of the day. I knew it was time to talk to the dean about quitting.

The dean seemed to understand my situation, but he did ask if I could stay until the end of the semester. I agreed to try. But when I went to the nurse's office to talk to her, she heard a rattle in my voice and urged me to get to a doctor right away. I went to a nearby doctor's office, but since he wasn't my primary doctor, he wouldn't see me. So I went home and called Renee, who lived in Oregon. Even over the phone she could hear the rattle and urged me to go to the emergency room. I took her advice, and as soon as I got there, I was quickly whisked into a little cubicle. The doctor assessed me and immediately had the paramedics transport me to UCLA, where I went straight into the ICU. I was very sick with pneumonia.

The hospital called Rob to come to the ICU. Later, he admitted that all the way to the hospital, he thought I had died. Renee flew down from Oregon. She had been working at the hospital in Hillsboro when Stacey, her husband, called her, saying she needed to go to California. He had already packed her bag and bought her a plane ticket, and he picked her up at the hospital and drove her immediately to the airport. My sister, too, arrived at the hospital. I knew I must be pretty sick for all of them to be there.

While in the ICU, I participated in a pet therapy program the hospital had instituted for patients in intensive care. The premise of the program was that stroking an animal has positive effects on people coping with physical or mental problems and helps reduce anxiety. To prepare me, the nurses first placed a large sheet over me. Then they brought a dog to me, who had been washed and dried three separate times. It was such a joy to have him sit on my lap and let me pet him. As far as I was concerned, this pet therapy worked.

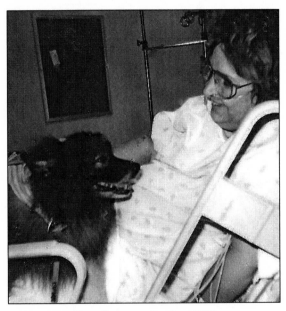

*Pet therapy in the ICU*

# *Chapter 16*

*O*nce I was home again, I tried to focus on taking care of myself. I had become far too weak to return to work. Renee suggested I move close to her in Oregon. I loved the idea of being near her and in a state that was so green. I flew to Oregon several times, ready to buy a home, but I couldn't find what I wanted. Renee, however, kept looking and exploring other options. She eventually found a retirement home near her. I trusted her judgment that it was a nice place and agreed to move in sight unseen.

I sold my home in California, packed up my furniture, and moved to Rosewood Park in Hillsboro. I lived only five minutes from Renee, and life was good. I so enjoyed being with my daughter and doing things with my grandchildren. When my grandson Colin came over, he would often ride his tricycle while I chased him around the building in my scooter. Renee and I also took the children to movies, parks, and to the ocean, but we especially liked to go shopping.

When my friend Rosemarie came to visit, we all went to the zoo. At that time, I was still able to stand a little. When it came time to leave the zoo, Renee and Rosemarie were trying to help me stand so that I could get back into her Blazer when my knees suddenly gave way. The only thing that kept me from falling was Renee's quick thinking as she positioned her knee in front of mine. That was the last day I was ever able to stand.

Obviously, I now needed more help, so I moved from the retirement side of Rosewood to the assisted living side, which catered to older, more incapacitated adults. Social and cultural programs and amenities fostered an easy way of life that I enjoyed. Bus trips to the ocean, wine-and-cheese parties, and the friendliness of the staff and residents made for a nice, easy existence.

The only drawback to my new arrangement was that I was in my fifties while all the other residents were much older. For instance, my dining partners, Marge and Oscar, were in their late eighties. Although they were older, they were still lots of fun and entertained me with many interesting stories from their youth. Marge and her parents had actually moved to Oregon from Minnesota by covered wagon. On their journey west, whenever they stopped at a town, her father would pull the back flap up from the covered wagon, revealing their piano. The townspeople were absolutely thrilled when her mother played the piano for them. When Marge and Oscar married, he bought her the first pair of shoes she had ever owned. The first house they bought cost five dollars. Stories like these kept me entertained for hours and drew me closer to my older friends.

One particular daily routine I especially looked forward to was attending Mass at the local Catholic Church, St. Elizabeth Ann Seton. It was a small church, and the people were very friendly. It didn't take long before I was very involved and assumed responsibility for organizing get-togethers for the new parishioners. For several years, I served on the pastoral council, an advisory board to the pastor.

The staff at Rosewood Park was more my age than were the residents, so I became friends with them too. We often went out together to clubs or events. But despite my friendship with the staff, it soon became rather depressing living with so many older residents. It seemed an ambulance and paramedics were there all the time. When my friend Marge died, I decided to move out into my own apartment.

A friend of mine, Mindy, helped me move into a two-bedroom apartment with beautiful flowers and a play area for my grandchildren, Colin and Chelsey. But only two years after I moved to Oregon, Renee and her family moved to Washington State. She wanted me to move with them, but because of Stacey's job, I was sure she would soon move from there as well. I didn't want to keep moving from place to place so decided to stay put.

My sister, her husband, and her friend Nancy arrived for a much-anticipated visit. We three women decided to drive out to the ocean, which was only an hour away. On the trip home, we had the unfortunate experience of hitting a deer. It dashed across the freeway so fast there was no way to avoid hitting it. Luckily, none of us were hurt, but my van did sustain quite a bit of damage.

We immediately called AAA, letting them know that I was handicapped and needed special assistance in getting back to Beaverton. They confidently assured us they could take care of me. As we were sitting on the side of the road waiting for AAA to arrive, a lady pulled over to see if we needed help. We assured her we were fine, but she insisted on staying, just to make sure.

After we had waited four hours, the tow truck finally arrived. During all that time, the lady kept insisting she would stay until the truck arrived, and it was a good thing she did! Despite their assurances, the company had made no provision for my disability, and it was impossible for me to get into the truck. The lady kindly offered to drive us back to Beaverton and during the drive told us a little about her life. Amazingly, she had been a secretary to Dr. Jonas Salk, the discoverer of the polio vaccine. Mary Jo and I were sure she was an angel in disguise.

# Chapter 17

When I went to the hospital with pneumonia again, I had no family nearby. It was an anxious, lonely time, so after being released from the hospital, I thought it best to move closer to relatives. Rob and his wife, Oanh, lived in Palmdale, California, and they asked me to live with them. To give me privacy and my own space, they transformed his garage into a lovely room for me. It had a beautiful window, a built-in closet, and even a small refrigerator.

It was so good to be with family, especially with their new baby, Katherine, who was born just four months after I moved in. Many times Rob would bring her downstairs, and they both would peek around the door to tell me good morning. Brittany, her sister, would have her breakfast and then stop in to talk to me before going to school. How I loved those visits! Rob's children, just like Renee's, loved my scooter. Each of my grandchildren has stood on the bar on the back and hung on while I motored around. When they were little, we pretended we were a train and would blow our imaginary horn. Katherine, now seven years old, still rides on it.

While living at Rob's, I learned to love Vietnamese food. I had never liked egg rolls until I ate the ones Oanh made. They were absolutely exceptional! Plus, the food she prepared was quite nutritious, keeping everyone healthy and slim.

I continued dealing with various health concerns, one of which was my heart. My cardiologist ordered a stress test, but because I could not actually physically exercise, I was given medicine to force my heart to work harder. The procedure was done under a local anesthetic, so after the test I was able to talk to the doctor while lying on the operating table. He informed me that 80 percent of one of my arteries was blocked, and he asked if I wanted a stent inserted. Of course, I said yes!

A year later, wanting my independence, I moved into my own apartment. I hired caregivers to help me in the mornings and evenings because I needed assistance in dressing and bathing. It was fun to putter around in my own kitchen again, and I was thankful I could still drive to daily Mass.

In April of 2005, I was admitted into Antelope Valley Hospital with pneumonia. I was very sick, and it was nineteen days before I was well enough to leave. Unable to stay home alone, I was transferred to a nursing home. At the nursing home, two patients occupied each room. My roommate had her own television to watch and family pictures hung on the wall. She had her own bedspread and made her side of the room as comfortable as possible. Her room had become her home.

I didn't want my side of the room to be too comfortable or like home. I was driven by another goal: I wanted to get out. My side of the room was bare, and I intended to keep it that way. My days were spent looking out the window or watching my roommate's television when it was on. I was in the nursing home for three weeks but don't remember much of that time. That is probably a blessing.

When I was finally allowed to return to my apartment, I had a hospital bed put into my living room. A physical therapist visited twice weekly to help me with exercises. Getting back to a fairly good functioning level was a slow process, but only three months later, I was admitted to the Lancaster Community Hospital—again with pneumonia. This time the nursing home stay lasted thirty days.

When I first went into the home, I wasn't even able to sit up on my own, so they placed me in a reclining chair near the nurses' station during the day. Every morning a nurse would come in around four or four-thirty to get me dressed and put me in my chair. Twice a week, I was taken to the shower at this early hour. This was not pleasant, since older people tend to get cold easily. At seven the new shift would come in and give me my breakfast. There were a few activities and exercises during the day, but most of the time I simply watched TV, longing for the day I could go home.

I went home weaker than the first time but still able to manage on my own with some help. But I was home no more than three weeks before I was back in the hospital again. This time, however, I was there for only six days. It seemed I couldn't completely get well. My apartment was so lovely, with lots of trees all around, but Renee hypothesized that the cool, damp climate probably encouraged the growth of mold and was the reason I couldn't get better.

I was out of the hospital for five days this time before I got very sick again. I knew I had to do something different; something was not right, and I needed answers. I asked Rob to pick me up and drive me to UCLA in Westwood, the hospital I had been going to since 1964. I was hopeful they could identify what was wrong with me and thus halt my rapid decline. On the way to the hospital, I was clear-headed and aware of everything, even to the point of telling Rob which exit to take. However, as soon as we arrived, that clarity vanished, and I have no memory of what took place after I passed through the emergency room doors.

When I finally began to gain some awareness, I thought I was in a tunnel about to be zapped with a Taser gun from all sides. I was so frightened that I couldn't breathe, and I was screaming inside my head, *If you're going to kill me, do it fast!* I started praying and exited the tunnel into a horrifying coldness—then nothing.

The next thing I knew I was in a hospital in Santa Monica. Renee and my grandchildren Chelsey and Colin were at my bedside. It upset me that the three of them had flown in from Minnesota because I wanted them to visit when we could go shopping together!

But everyone had gathered at my bedside: Rob and his family, my sister from Idyllwild, my grandson Robbie, and my nephew Jim and his wife, Janet. I knew I must be in pretty bad shape.

What really stunned me, however, was the fact that I was totally paralyzed. I couldn't fathom what had happened to me, but I didn't want to be paralyzed again, like I had been so many years before. I couldn't move my arms or legs at all, so I was unable to push the call button when I needed something. The nurses looked around and finally located a flat call button that I could press by exerting just a little pressure with the heel of my right hand.

Two men came in every four hours, day and night, to turn me from one side to the other so as to prevent bed sores. When it was almost time for them to come, I'd anxiously watch the clock. It felt so wonderful when they changed my position.

The doctors couldn't figure out what was wrong with me. They did test me for polio, but thank God the test came back negative. I couldn't imagine having to go through that again! Then I was tested for the Guillain-Barre syndrome. This is a rather rare inflammatory disorder of the immune system and results in an attack upon the nerves. In many cases, it's triggered by a viral infection, and a procedure called plasmapheresis is the prescribed therapy.

The purpose of plasmapheresis is to remove toxic substances from the blood. The basic procedure consists of removing the blood, separating the blood cells from plasma, and returning the blood cells to the body's circulation. The process involves IV administration every other day for a total of ten days. A large board with eighteen IVs was set up next to my bed. A nurse turned one IV on and then off, then another on and off. She continued this process for the next four hours while recording extensive notes. Nothing happened; I still couldn't move, so they canceled the procedure.

Twenty-four hours later, however, my right arm began to move. With that encouraging sign, the doctors decided to continue plasmapheresis for the next ten days. Despite everything that was going on in my body, I wasn't concerned or frightened. I accepted the moment the way it was, a trait that has always been part of me and has seen me through many a trial.

I was then transferred to Brotman Rehabilitation Center in Santa Monica, and for the next fourteen days, I endured intense physical therapy. The therapists attempted to position me upright in a standing machine, but my legs crumbled. Additionally, my neck muscles were paralyzed, which meant I was unable to eat regular food. Although I had been taken off the IVs, the only thing I could eat was pureed food. If the hospital was serving eggs and biscuits for breakfast, then those two ingredients were blended together for my meal. It was horrid! What a relief when I could eat regular food again!

Four weeks after entering the hospital, I was home. Although I was nearly back to my pre-hospital strength, I never regained the original strength of my good leg. When I got in my van to drive, I couldn't even lift my good leg high enough to reach the gas or brake pedal. Crushed, I realized I would never be able to drive again.

After giving it some thought, I determined that if I had to go into the hospital again, I would move out of my apartment. Maybe Renee was right about mold in the apartment as the cause of my physical ailments. With that in mind, I went about my life, slowly gaining strength until four months later the all-too-familiar pattern repeated itself: I was back in the Lancaster Community Hospital with pneumonia!

During this stay, I experienced a rather scary incident. I shared a room with another woman, and one day she asked me to call the nurse for her, since her call bell wasn't working. Happy to oblige, I rang the bell, and the next thing I knew I was in the ICU and intubated. When the nurse had entered the room, she quickly observed that I had stopped breathing so administered CPR and rushed me to the ICU. I was grateful for her life-saving action, but my ribs were sore for days.

Shortly after this episode, my niece Susan came to see me and asked, "When you stopped breathing, did you see the white light everyone talks about?"

"No, I didn't see the light, but I did see terrorists climbing in the window," I replied. We both got a big laugh out of that, but when it was happening, it was truly frightening. Susan and I concluded that I must have been given some rather potent drugs.

Days later I went into the nursing home again, and while I was there, I decided it was time to move from my apartment, just like I had said I would do if I had to go to the hospital again. My caregiver and

I went out every afternoon looking for a new place until we found just the right one. Thus begins the current stage of my life.

# *Chapter 18*

*T*oday I live in an "over fifty-five and active" complex. I have a two-bedroom apartment with sunshine streaming in my east windows and onto my patio on the west. No more cool and shady apartment, but no more damp and mold! Three years have passed since I moved here, and I have not been back into the hospital. Obviously, my daughter was right in her assessment.

Every year Rob, Oanh, and their kids visit Oanh's parents in San Jose at Christmastime, but I stay home. Several years ago when I was still driving, I was getting ready for Mass on Christmas morning. Before I left, I called Renee to wish her a happy Christmas. We chatted casually for a bit, and then Renee apologized for being late in sending my gift. But, she explained, she was paying extra for UPS to deliver it on Christmas Day. I told her that it wasn't necessary to do that; it was perfectly fine if the present arrived a few days late.

Thinking no more about it, I attended Mass then returned home. I decided to call Renee again, but Stacey answered the phone and said she was in the shower and would call me back a little later. A few hours passed with no phone call, but again I didn't think much about it. A little later, there was a knock on the door, and a deep voice boomed, "UPS, merry Christmas!" *I guess Renee went ahead and sent the present,* I thought as I made my way to the door, wondering why it was so important to her to have it delivered on Christmas Day.

As I opened the door, I was greeted with, "Surprise, Mom! Merry Christmas! Hope you like your present!" and there stood Renee. She was my Christmas package—and such a wonderful surprise! Little did I know that when I had called to speak to her earlier, she was actually in an airplane on her way to me. She stayed only two days, but what a wonderful two days they were!

On a day-to-day basis, my life moves in a predictable routine. A caregiver arrives in the morning at eight to get me out of bed, help me dress, and cook my meals. In the evening, she makes dinner and then helps me back into bed before she leaves at seven. She helps me into bed by lifting my bad leg and holding it up while I push against my chair with my good leg, and then, with arms stretched back and locked, I slowly scoot back until I'm completely on the bed.

Since I'm sitting all day, she exercises my arms and legs at night to keep them strong and supple. It feels wonderful, and I look forward to this part of my day. I have a sleep-number bed whose height I can adjust, so I can sit up and watch television when I'm alone at night. Like anything else, however, it is subject to malfunctions, which I discovered one night when it deflated and paramedics had to rescue me! Before going to sleep, I ready my oxygen and my BiPap, which I use every night.

Thank God, I am still independent enough to live on my own. Once in a while, I do have to call Rob late at night for help, but he never seems to mind. He always so kindly responds to my requests and says, "That's okay, Mom. I expect it; don't worry about it."

Katherine, my granddaughter, visits me often, which is a great delight to me. If she has homework, she must do it before we play.

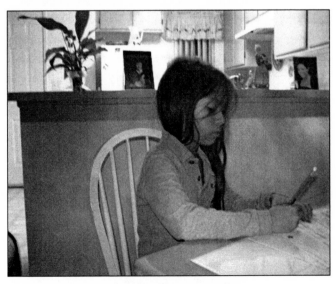

*Katherine concentrating*

We do lots of different things together. Sometimes she waters my garden, and other times we play games and do crafts. But if I give her a choice and ask her what she wants to do, the answer is always the same: "I want to bake."

Treasuring this special time with my granddaughter, I sit in my chair at the end of the kitchen cabinet. Together we read the recipe for whatever we're baking, which is always from scratch. Katherine gets out the electric mixer, measures the ingredients, sifts flour—everything that's needed for the recipe. Sometimes the dough gets too stiff, so she sits on the floor to have more leverage to stir it. I touch absolutely nothing.

Because she has just had her seventh birthday, I feel she's too young to put anything into a hot oven. So we prepare the recipe but don't turn the oven on until we have placed whatever we're baking inside. It may not be the most traditional way of doing things, but it works just fine for us.

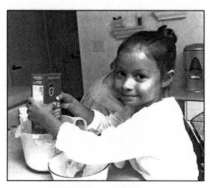

*The busy baker*

It's such a joy for me to be a grandma and involved in my grandchildren's lives. I'm able to spend more time with Katherine than I was ever able to do with my children, but I suppose that's what grandmas do!

And Katherine is good company in many ways. Like a little mother hen, she watches to see if I need anything. If my leg falls from my wheelchair, she takes both her little hands and lifts it back into place. She's very serious about doing it just right so it doesn't hurt me. We all refer to Katherine as our miracle child because she was conceived eight years after Rob had a vasectomy. She was meant to be born!

Brittany, Katherine's older sister, comes over when I need help. Every time she leaves, she always makes the same sweet offer: "Call me if you need me." She recently graduated from high school and is now enrolled in art school in San Diego. I'm very proud of her, like I am of all my grandchildren.

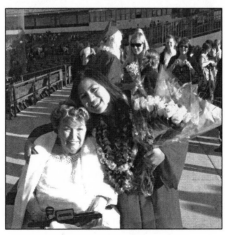

***Brit's Graduation Day***

# Chapter 19

*I* don't go out of the complex often, but when I do, I use my van. Since my legs are too weak to drive, my caregiver drives me. In the last four years, however, I've had horrendous problems with my van. But the van is fifteen years old, so I guess I shouldn't be too surprised!

I bought the handicapped-converted van when I was still working; my payments were 450 dollars a month, and the loan was for ten years. It was very difficult to make those payments, but I did and finally paid the van off. By that time, however, problems were popping up. The most difficult and exasperating problem concerned the van ramp and door. Every time the door didn't work, I had to find someone to drive the van the sixty miles to the auto-repair shop that worked on handicapped conversions.

On two occasions, the door for my ramp wouldn't open, trapping me in my van until paramedics could get me out. Since I no longer drive and don't need the automatic door opener, the remedy was fairly simple:

I had the door fixed so it would open manually. But life is seldom as simple as we hope, and I soon had trouble with the manual door. Recently, as my caregiver was opening the door, it partially fell off!

One particular problem with the van happened when my caregiver was driving me to the doctor's office in Palmdale. Suddenly we heard an earsplitting pop and thought we had blown a tire, but the trouble was actually with the air bags under the van. These bags allow my van to move up and down so that I can access it. When I press the remote, the van lowers closer to the ground and the ramp comes down. It is an absolutely essential function for me, as you can imagine.

When this happened, Rob was out of town and unavailable to help. We called the public bus for the handicapped, only to be told that I had to make an appointment the day before. This was clearly an emergency, but they still wouldn't pick me up. My only option was to ride inside the van as it sat on top of the flatbed of the towing truck. That was one wild, bumpy ride! To make matters worse, it was over one hundred degrees that day. Although it was against the law to let me stay in the van, the tow-truck driver realized my dilemma and had compassion on me.

There's another way the problems with the van have affected my life. When I moved back from Oregon to California, I began attending daily Mass at St. Mary Catholic Church. One morning Father Cyprian Carlos asked me to read the second reading, which is always from the New Testament. Since I could not maneuver the steps leading to the altar, the sacristan set up a music stand with the Bible in place and handed me a microphone. Soon I was reading regularly at Sunday Mass.

When a new church was built in the parish, they built a ramp behind the altar. This allowed me to read on the altar itself. The sacristan could open the door at the top of the ramp, and I could easily roll onto the altar. For the last three years, I was privileged to read the second reading every other Sunday. I loved trying to convey the meaning of the sacred words, and I loved being active and involved in the church. Unfortunately, since I've had so much trouble with my van, I eventually had to switch to a church closer to my home. I knew it was a necessary move, but it was an emotionally difficult one because that church congregation had become like family.

# *Chapter 20*

*R*enee thought we should all get together as a family and started making arrangements for our first family reunion at Lake Arrowhead, California. In December 2007, she rented a handicapped-accessible cabin at the lake for the following August. Her cousins Sue and John both live at the lake, and all the rest of the family lives nearby. In August Renee and her daughter, Chelsey, flew down from Minneapolis so they could drive me to the reunion in my van. I was very excited for the chance to see my relatives and to take such an excursion. This was the first time since my many hospital stays that I left Lancaster and emerged from my cocoon.

Prior to the trip, I had the van checked to make sure everything was working properly. Before driving to Lake Arrowhead, we first drove to San Diego to see my former mother-in-law and then went on to visit my sister in Idyllwild. Mary Jo's home sits perched in the mountains at sixty-three hundred feet and has so many steps it's impossible for me to stay with her.

Hoping to find a place for me nearby, she checked with several cabin rentals in the area and located one with only a few steps. Years before I bought a folding metal ramp, and with it in place, I zipped over the steps and into the cabin.

What a difference a change of scenery can make! It was so refreshing to be in the mountains with the smell of the pine trees and the wonderful mountain air. It was just what I needed. After being in and out of the hospital so many times in the last few years, it was absolutely wonderful to feel like a normal person again.

I was so grateful to be with Renee on this long trip. Not only did she have to do all the driving, but she also had to help me dress and undress and help me in and out of bed. Furthermore, I'm not able to use any public restrooms, even handicapped ones. I require special accommodations wherever I go because my needs are different from most. Renee willingly assumed the task of helping me and always does so with such grace and love.

The next day, we took the National Scenic Byway to Lake Arrowhead, which affords a spectacular view of the surrounding mountains and the Los Angeles basin. After entering the national forest, the four-lane road quickly gains elevation, reaching four thousand feet after only eight miles. Staying in the slow lane, we faced the outside. It was a long, long way to the bottom, I noticed, and since I don't do well with heights, I was rather nervous but tried not to show it. As the driver, Renee was understandably very tense, but after many tight horseshoe curves, we made it to the rental cabin, all in one piece.

The cabin was located down a very steep incline, so my van was pointed downward when I tried to get out. This made the ramp from my van sit at an angle, which tilted my scooter. Renee held one side of the scooter so I wouldn't fall over and managed to get me down the ramp and to the walkway leading to the cabin. However, although the cabin was supposed to be handicapped-accessible, there was a huge bump in the concrete that made forward progress impossible. We got out my metal ramp again, but we decided it was too hazardous for us to try it alone. When my nephews and son arrived, we came up with a plan. Because the concrete bump was lopsided, my legs were tied to the scooter so they wouldn't fall off it when my nephews tilted my chair. It took one nephew in back, one on each side, and my son in front steering the scooter controls to get me to the cabin. But we made it!

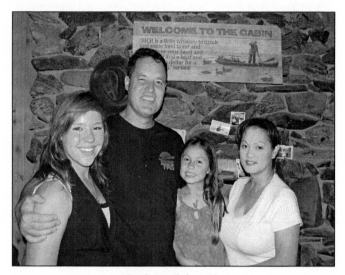

*Rob and family*

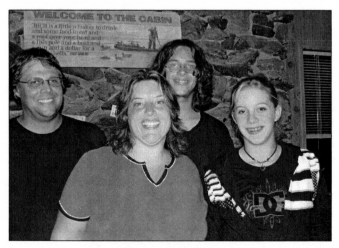

*Renee and fami*

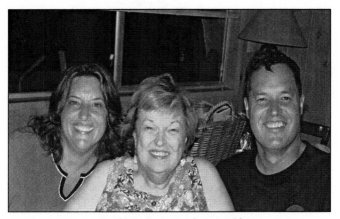

*Rob Renee and myself*

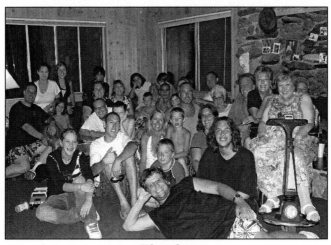

*The clan*

The next day we all went to the lake, all thirty-five of us. We braved the big bump again, and I sat on a hillside and watched as everyone went swimming or boating. Oanh and my sister sat with me. It was good to watch my two granddaughters getting to know each other. Heather is from Montana and Chelsey lives in Minnesota, but our reunion gave them a chance to meet.

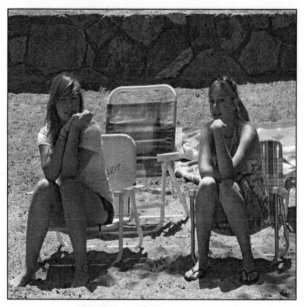

*Getting to know you…...*

A side note about Chelsey: She once wrote an essay about me for her class. I had no idea I had made such an impression on her. The following is an excerpt from her school's award winning essay titled "My Amazing Grandma."

I love spending time with my grandma. We also talk, play games, and we always go shopping together. When I was little, I would ride on the back of her wheelchair. . . . My grandma is great, and she has taught me so much. It is so much fun having her around. I think it is amazing what she has been through.

I was so touched when reading her essay that I decided to use one of her words, "amazing," as part of the title of my book. I have indeed had an amazing life, but it has been full of amazing people every step of the way. I have a special thank you for my teenage grandson Colin's help on my computer. When in need of computer help always call a teenager.

Back to the reunion: The time to leave came all too soon, and we maneuvered the bump one last time. I made it to the van with no incident, but when Rob tried to back up the van, it wouldn't go into reverse. He tried a number of times, and it just wouldn't budge. Out I came from the van, and we had to decide how to transport me. Susan called the tow service to take my van down the mountain to my home, and we used a board to get me into Stacey's rental car. I hadn't been in a regular car for many years. What a smooth ride! My van hits all the bumps hard and jolts my back, so it was such a pleasure to ride in a regular car again.

# *Chapter 21*

*T*oday I'm back in my apartment, playing Mexican train dominoes with my friends. I'm staying engaged in life and waiting for the next episode to begin. Always willing to break out of my cocoon, I enjoy life. To be sure, challenges and difficulties are there, but joy and love are also present— and in greater abundance.

When my daughter organized the family reunion, she e-mailed each person about me and said, "As you know, this is all for her, so whatever makes her happy makes me happy." That's the kind of daughter she is. She still calls me almost every day. In fact, we talk so much that she says that when I die, she's going to put my cell phone in my casket so she can call it to hear my voice. I'd better keep my phone well charged!

I've been blessed by my son as well as my daughter. He wrote the following poem, "Courage," about me.

Courage

The measure of one's courage should not be judged alone
by how tall a mountain is… but also by how tall
was the mountain to the one who climbed it.
—Robert F Dieguez

Yes, I have climbed mountains that sometimes seemed insurmountable, but I could not have done it without the help of so many wonderful people. Although they call me amazing, I think they are amazing too, and the richness of my life would not be possible without them. Amazing people, an amazing God, and the amazing courage that only He can provide have blessed me with a truly remarkable, amazing life!

LaVergne, TN USA
28 May 2010
184422LV00001B/16/P